Little Sugar Addicts

Little Sugar Addicts

End the Mood Swings,
Meltdowns, Tantrums, and
Low Self-Esteem
In Your Child Today

KATHLEEN DesMAISONS, Ph.D.

 THREE RIVERS PRESS · NEW YORK

Published by Three Rivers Press, New York, New York.
Member of the Crown Publishing Group, a division of
Random House, Inc.
www.crownpublishing.com

THREE RIVERS PRESS and the Tugboat design are registered trademarks of Random House, Inc.

Printed in the United States of America

Design by Helene Berinsky

Library of Congress Cataloging-in-Publication Data
DesMaisons, Kathleen.
   Little sugar addicts : end the mood swings, meltdowns, tantrums, and low self-esteem in your child today /
Kathleen DesMaisons.
      Includes bibliographical references.
   1. Sugar-free diet.   2. Sugar—Physiological effect.   3. Affective disorders in children—Diet therapy.   4. Children—Nutrition—Psychological aspects.   I. Title.
   RM237.85.D467 2004
   641.5'638—dc22   2003028178

ISBN 1-4000-5164-9

10 9 8 7 6 5 4 3

First Edition

To Mother, who taught me that children come first

ACKNOWLEDGMENTS

This book comes from the dialogue with the members of our Web community at www.radiantrecovery.com. The insight and lived experience of the parents and children who talked so openly and deeply about their journey have made the solution in this book a living dialogue. I am deeply grateful to be a part of their healing. I am also grateful to the generous volunteers who make the community possible. Their dedication and commitment allow us to directly support tens of thousands every day.

The vision and enthusiasm of Becky Cabaza at Three Rivers Press made it a joy to write the book. Thanks to Mary Ann Naples for her belief in the concept and for finding the perfect editor for the job. A great team for a fun collaboration!

CONTENTS

Little Sugar Addicts

Introduction

Do you have a smart, creative, compassionate child who is also spacey, inattentive, cranky, and sometimes obnoxious? Does your child have unexpected meltdowns or temper tantrums that make no sense to you? Is your child getting tubby and suffering at school because of it? Has your doctor told you that your child is prediabetic? Have you put your son on medication for ADD?

I know that you really care for your child and that you know something is not right. The contradictions simply make no sense. Your child can be sweet and loving—or fearful, cranky, out of control, moody, depressed, or destructive. Yet this same child has moments of being enchanting, funny, gifted, tender, compassionate, loving, and creative. There are moments when he touches you deeply—and times when you would like to trade him in for a new model! The pain you feel at seeing your gentle and loving child turn willful, frightened, or out of control is beyond words. The rage you feel in the midst of the power struggles terrifies you.

1

Sometimes it feels as if you are living with a split personality. The changes in behavior simply make no sense. You wonder what is behind it and you simply do not know what to do. You feel as if everyone has something to say—and much of it is aimed at you. If *you* would just get your child straightened out, things would be okay. You *want* to be a good parent. You work hard at it, but you are tired down to your very bones. You cannot imagine struggling with one more fight to get chores done, to finish homework, to not eat junk, to get to school on time.

You don't want to struggle like this. You want your child to be happy and well adjusted. You begin to wonder if drugs are the answer. Maybe you have tried medications, and they didn't work or didn't work for long. You wonder about diet. You have tried making "healthy" meals, but your children refuse to eat them. They announce, "I am not eating *that!*" and stomp away. You have bargained with them, you have pleaded, you have prayed—and things have not changed.

I am convinced that what you are experiencing is a function of your child's biochemistry and diet. It is not about your parenting skills or some flaw in your child's character. It is not a psychological disorder. Your child may be sugar sensitive. A biochemical imbalance can create all sorts of negative behavior in your child. This is *not* your fault. It is not your child's fault. Sugar sensitivity is an inherited biochemical condition that affects how the brain and body function. Mood swings, erratic behavior, inability to concentrate, low self-esteem, fatigue, crankiness, and being overweight are all connected and can all be driven by the biochemical imbalance of untreated sugar sensitivity. These behaviors are *not* a result of your parenting skills.

What and when your children eat creates the contradictions you see in them. If a sugar sensitive child skips meals, eats late, has a lot of sugar, eats refined foods, or doesn't get the right nutrients, she will be erratic, moody, unable to concentrate, chubby, cranky, dramatic, funny, wildly energetic, temperamental, or spacey. The program I will outline for you is not about taking your child off of all sugars or avoiding food additives; it is about designing a food program that heals the reason for the problems. It is about going right to the cause rather than trying to deal with the symptoms. It is about healing biochemistry by changing the food.

Changing your child's food will have an effect beyond anything you can imagine. The program I will outline is based on very specific science and has been tested for many years. It has already had an extraordinary impact on thousands and thousands of families.

It's like getting the big-kid equivalent of the "easy baby." You know, the one that smiles, sleeps well, plays well, goes everywhere, and rarely fusses. Steady food and steady routine bring out the easy kid. Even our high-energy, intense kids are closer to their "easy" selves.

Connie

How It All Began

Why do I care about you and your child? How do I have the expertise to show you the way out of this dilemma? How do I know what works and what doesn't? Let me give you a little background so you can get a sense of where I am coming from.

I started examining the idea of sugar sensitivity about

fifteen years ago. I was running an alcoholism treatment center and looking for ways to improve treatment. It didn't seem right that only 20 percent of our clients were able to get sober and stay sober. I started reading scientific journals and came across an obscure article that made a one-line reference to a connection between sugar and alcoholism. It grabbed my attention.

Intuitively, I knew there was something to this idea. I had stopped drinking when I was in my early twenties, but my relationship to sugar had been so much like my clients' relationship to alcohol that it shocked me. I would lie about or hide my use of sugar, I couldn't stop having it, and my day was planned around when I could get my sugar fix. I had terrible mood swings, and the changes in my personality during the course of the day confused me.

I had changed my diet and discovered the strong connection between what I ate and how I felt. That article started me thinking about the biochemistry of diet. I began asking my alcoholic clients what they ate. I learned that none of them ate breakfast, and most ate lots of sugar and refined carbohydrates. None of them had regular meals, and very few ate protein at every meal. Their eating habits were quite similar—and quite poor.

So I designed a food plan to support their recovery from alcoholism and began to include it as a major aspect of treatment. My clients learned to eat meals at regular and consistent times, to eat protein at each meal, to stop eating sugars, and to make some other important adjustments to their food *before* attempting to stop drinking. Adding this dietary component to treatment had remarkable results. Our success rate climbed to 92 percent. That is, 92 percent of the alcoholics who graduated from our program were sober and stayed that way. As the clients continued doing the food program and staying sober, they reported consistent and striking changes in their behavior and moods. They were clear and focused, and they had more energy and increased self-esteem. They were able to problem-solve and use other resources to support their sobriety. Their relationships improved. They got jobs or promotions. The changes were beyond anything we expected in early sobriety from alcoholism.

These results—a success rate increasing from 20 to 92 percent—were astonishing. I knew I was on to something big, but I was not sure how the biochemistry worked. I had seen the change in myself and observed it in others, but I did not know why it was happening. I made the life-changing decision to go back to school to get a Ph.D. and sort out the science behind what I had seen and experienced. So I sold my house, gave up my position as director of the clinic, moved into a one-room apartment, and committed my life to understanding the scientific facts.

I learned that there is powerful scientific evidence for the fact that certain people are very, very vulnerable to the effects of sugar. Sugar acts like a drug in the body—it affects the same brain chemicals that heroin and morphine do. After poring over thousands of scientific journals, I began to formulate my theory of sugar sensitivity. Certain people, I realized, are born with an imbalance in three parts of their brain and body chemistry: they have low serotonin (the chemical that "quiets" the brain and helps with saying no), low beta-endorphin (the brain's own "painkiller"), and volatile blood sugar. These three disturbances set them up to react profoundly to the druglike effects of sugar. And their sugar sensitive brain chemistry leads them into addictive patterns and more and more compromised eating. You will read more about these three concerns and how they fit together in Chapter 1.

I also began to see why changing the food could change the behavior of these individuals in such a powerful way. I saw that "doing the food" could heal the brain and body chemistry disturbances and restore the sugar sensitive person to a balanced and functional life. My studies and ensuing doctorate provided me with the scientific basis for explaining the huge changes that had happened with the alcoholics in my clinic.

Sharing the Solution

I needed to bring this story to the public—the results were too powerful to keep hidden. In 1998 I wrote *Potatoes Not Prozac*, a catchy title that targeted folks who were being told that the solution to their depression, mood swings, and low self-esteem was antidepressants. Although the title emphasized the idea of using potatoes to boost serotonin, the book presented my entire theory of sugar sensitivity. It introduced the idea that sugar sensitivity is a biochemical condition, not a character flaw, and that it can be treated by a change in diet.

People were excited by the book! They wanted to understand how to implement the ideas. *The Sugar Addict's Total Recovery Program* followed in 2000, as a road map for them. At the same time I set up a website at www. radiantrecovery.com to create a community for people doing the food program. The site provided a way for people from all over to talk with one another about their food. What started as a quiet dialogue of a few hundred people has since turned into an ongoing tutorial and discussion on healing for thousands and thousands of sugar sensitive men and women.

Sugar sensitive people from every corner of the world met one another online and began to talk. Twenty-five million hits to the website told me I was on to something even bigger than I had originally imagined. At first most of those corresponding were middle-aged women who had tried every diet in the world and were ready for a plan that actually *worked*. Then younger women started visiting the site and joining the discussion. They came to heal their own sugar sensitivity. Pretty soon they started to see a connection between diet and their children's behavior. They started asking, "What shall we do with our children, Kathleen?"

So I set up a forum for parents to talk with one another. The parents started sharing. We talked, we explored. At first it seemed like a smart idea to simply take the Seven Steps I had created for adults and adapt them to kids. It sounded pretty straightforward. All we needed to do was to support the parents in getting their kids off sugar: just do the steps, and things would be fine.

This was both simplistic and naïve. Huge problems emerged. The first, of course, was that the children did not think there was a problem with how they ate. Second, they were not in any way interested in taking sweet things out of their diets. They had not experienced the self-reflection and the years of struggle that Mom had experienced prior to starting healing her own sugar sensitivity. They had no personal motivation to change, and they were very attached to their "drugs."

In addition, many of the women's spouses and partners thought making dietary changes was either silly or a really bad idea: "Why would you want to make the kids give up something that gives them such pleasure?" Often huge resistance came from Daddy. Daddy loves ice cream. Daddy loves taking the kids out for pizza and Cokes on Friday night. Or Daddy lives in another house, and whatever efforts Mom makes with the kids' eating during the week goes down the drain on the weekends.

The schools and teachers, too, were an obstacle. They were steeped in the idea of treats as reward, sugar as celebration, sugar as respite. Cupcakes for parties, candy for Halloween, Coke machines in the cafeteria, and lunch provided by fast-food vendors combined to make a powerful force against changing kids' eating habits.

Then, of course, there were grandparents, aunties, cousins, and friends. The idea of keeping kids off sugar and having them eat only healthy food sounded good, but it was a daunting task. Family members rebelled or got frustrated with it. It seemed for a while as if we were just making things worse: we were adding to the power struggle, creating more fuel for upset in families that were already fatigued and volatile.

Changing the kids' diets was a great idea, but it brought up so many problems! So my online community and I focused on just changing Mom. We said, "Don't try to get your kids on the program yet, just do it yourself. Put on your own oxygen mask before helping others. Learn the nuances of the program, do the steps, do the food, watch what is happening with your body and your emotions. Don't worry about the kids right now."

To our surprise and delight, as Mom made changes, the kids got interested. The kids saw that Mom was eating differently and saw her behavior change drastically. They remembered her mood swings, her unpredictability, her

fatigue, her anger, her forgetting, her not keeping promises. They may have never talked about it, but they knew.
And now they were noticing that Mom was getting relaxed and funny. They noticed no more yelling, no more
tears; they noticed that doing fun things together was becoming a part of their routine.

In this way, their little brains registered the connection
between food and behavior. Of course, they were still not
at all excited about the idea of giving up sugar themselves.
Neither was Dad. But Mom took baby steps: she started
with insisting on breakfast with protein. That didn't seem
too bad to the kids. Yes, they could manage a protein
shake in the morning before school. And so it went, each
baby step building on previous baby steps. Major changes
started to happen. The baby steps accumulated. The kids
were eating differently. Their behavior started to change.
Things shifted: instead of just Mom doing her thing, the
kids began to buy in. They started getting excited and par-
ticipating. They began problem-solving together. The family became an oasis of sanity. In effect, they got steady and
stable together and started to figure out how to deal with
the outside world of craziness and sugar addiction.

Kids Take the Lead

These changes happened slowly. After a year, parents were
sending in amazing stories about how their children were
teaching those around them. The kids wanted to talk with
one another, so we formed an online club through our
website. They started sharing pancake recipes and talking
about applesauce and peanut butter. They shared about
their sugar-free birthday parties. They talked about how

to deal with going to Dad's house for the weekend. They figured out a time that allowed children from Perth, Australia, to talk with children from Boston, Denver, and Surrey, England. The kids were funny, outrageous, creative, and little geniuses at problem-solving!

> *I live in England too! It is nice to know there are other people who can't have sugar. When I eat sugar, I feel grumpy and I get cross easily and then I feel sad. It makes me feel like I am on another planet on my own and my skin goes all itchy and bumpy. If I eat a little bit, I want to eat more and more and then I get more grumpy.*
> Lucy

Their combined energy and wisdom were so powerful it took my breath away. These were the very same kids whose parents had described them as

the most stubborn, defiant, frustrating [kids] I have ever known.

They weren't in counseling, they didn't have new parents or grandparents, their schools hadn't changed, the media and advertising hadn't changed, but the kids *had*. Doing the food was transforming them.

Had the parents been struggling to make the changes in their family alone, in isolation, the steps toward success would have seemed so tiny that they would never have been noticed. But the reports shared on the website slowly wove a tapestry that showed us how profound the change was. An image here, a color there, a few stitches on the far side, and a powerful picture emerged.

This past weekend was Yom Kippur, the Jewish holiday. My husband and daughters and I were having dinner together Sunday night. I had baked an apple cake for dessert for the others. It is a traditional dessert this time of year for our family.

So, Eddie cuts himself and the girls each a small piece that they all enjoy, and then he cuts himself another piece when Lindsey breaks out into song! "Too much sugar, too much sugar, too much sugar for my dad," sung to the tune of "Found a Peanut." We were cracking up because "too much sugar" sounded like meshugie, *which in Yiddish means too crazy! How fitting.*

Gail

The positive change I had seen in the adults doing the program was even more powerful for the children. Children's bodies are far more responsive to dietary intervention. They bounce back more quickly from the depleting effects of sugar. They want to heal and flourish. Once the process takes hold and the child buys in to the relationship between food and feelings, and between food and behavior, there is no stopping.

Last night we had company for dinner. My nephew and brother were drinking diet soda. My daughter Kayla went into how they were messing up their brains! She was relentless! So finally one of them asked, "How exactly does it mess up my brain?" Her reply: "I forget but believe me it does." She learned that at the first Kid's Chat. I doubt she will ever touch the diet soda. She told me later that she needs to find out the exact way it messes up your brain so she can call Uncle Howard and tell him.

Gail

A child's natural curiosity and excitement about making connections is a powerful ally in the process. We discovered that the key to kids changing their food is *not* having the parents make them change but having the kids experience the relationship between what they eat and how they feel. Once the children make the connection of food → feelings → behavior, they will take it and run with it.

The biochemical solution of this diet is incredibly simple. Changing your child's food can give you back his sweet and loving side. Changing the food can help her focus, contribute to weight loss, alter blood sugar levels, eliminate mood swings, and defuse rage.

When my child is getting "low," she becomes the most stubborn human being on the face of the earth. On the other hand if I keep her belly filled up with good food, she is very good-natured, easygoing, and has an awesome sense of humor.

Jennifer

Changing your child's food can transform the power struggle into playful problem-solving. More than counseling, more than behavior therapy or boot camp, and more than drugs, changing what your child eats will provide a solid foundation for any other intervention you want to try. Let me help you understand sugar sensitivity and how it affects you and your family. You will see what powerful medicine food can be. I will teach you a step-by-step process for making changes that will work, and together we will create the "baby steps" to heal yourself and your family. You are not alone. You did not cause this problem; it is not your fault. And it *can* be healed. Read the whole book carefully, even the last chapter. Study it, use it, try out the recipes in the back. Follow the steps, and get back the child you love so much.

1

Is Your Child Sugar Sensitive?

If you are reading this book, you may intuitively feel that you have a sugar sensitive child. But how can you know for sure? We have no blood test yet that will tell you. What we do have, however, is a solid list of clues that has been developed over a long time and with a lot of input from parents just like you. Sugar sensitivity affects behavior, health, and emotions. Let's go through each one and see how your child fits the profile. Whether he is a toddler or she is a teen, most of these questions will apply.

Let's look first at your child's **behavior**:

☐ Does your child ask for sweet foods all the time?
☐ Does your child have unexpected meltdowns that turn into tantrums or tears?
☐ Is your child impulsive?
☐ Does your child have a very short fuse?
☐ Is your child wildly dramatic and goofy?
☐ Is your child restless and in motion all the time?

☐ Is your child known as a motormouth?

☐ Does your child have a hard time paying attention?

☐ Does your child lock into a task for a long time and forget to do anything else?

And check your child's **health:**

☐ Does your child have lots of allergies?

☐ Does your child still wet the bed?

☐ Does your child have persistent ear infections?

☐ Is your child overweight?

☐ Does your child come home from school exhausted?

☐ Has your child been diagnosed with diabetes?

☐ Has your child been diagnosed with ADD or ODD?

Finally, and perhaps most important, are the **emotional** clues:

☐ Does your child cry at the drop of a hat?

☐ Does your child go from being absolutely charming to pouting and being moody?

☐ Does your child have low self-esteem even though he or she is smart, skilled, and capable?

☐ Does your child feel alone, isolated, not a part of the in-crowd at school or in the playground?

If you checked three or more boxes from all the lists combined, you are reading the right book. Your child will benefit from a change in diet. If you checked many boxes, do not be alarmed—the more you checked, the more dramatic will be the results you get by changing what and when your child eats. You may have simply assumed that you have a moody child, or a little goofball who bounces around with a motormouth turned on. You may have figured these things were just a part of your child's personality or personal style and never considered that they have a biochemical basis and are connected. The truth is, *all* of these symptoms can be rooted in your child's biochemistry. The degree to which your child displays them is very connected to what and when she eats. You may be stunned at the positive changes in your child's behavior as you change the food.

Perhaps you have already made the connection between sugar and hyperactivity, but the idea of creating a sugar-free household is simply beyond your imagination. And if you are sugar sensitive yourself, you may have your own issues to resolve. You may feel like an inadequate parent because your children are so moody or mouthy. Sometimes you may join your children in evening treats to help contain the pain and complexity of your feelings. *Little Sugar Addicts* will show you the way out. You will recover both your own joy in parenting and your child's happiness. You will learn the skills to transform your family in a kind and practical way. The mood swings and meltdowns will disappear. Self-esteem will skyrocket, and the entire family will start having fun.

My kids and I enjoy each other more. We have more fun and want to spend time together. They don't fight with each other, they are better at problem solving, and don't expect me to do everything for them. I always "knew" what wonderful, creative, intelligent, and caring kids I have. Now I "see" those traits every day.

Vicki

Let's go on to learn about what sugar sensitivity is and what you can do about it. *Sugar sensitivity* is the term I coined in my doctoral thesis to describe a physical condition that includes three key imbalances: a volatile blood sugar response to sugar and simple carbohydrates, low serotonin, and low beta-endorphin. If you have an alcoholic, depressed, or overweight parent or grandparent, you may have inherited this biochemistry. If you are sugar sensitive, what and when you eat makes a huge difference in how you feel and act. A diet of erratic meals, high sugar, and lots of refined carbohydrates will create havoc. It will foster the behaviors that are in the diagnostic profile I just gave you.

The Biology of Sugar Sensitivity

Let's talk about the biochemistry of sugar sensitivity and how all the pieces fit together. Imagine a stool with three legs, each with its own name: *blood sugar, serotonin,* and *beta-endorphin.*

Blood Sugar

Let's look at the first leg: blood sugar. This leg is critical for sugar sensitive children, so listen carefully to the story. Normally, when you eat foods made up of carbohydrates (sugars and starches), your blood sugar rises and your body releases a hormone called insulin. Insulin helps your cells draw sugar from your bloodstream to use as fuel. This is a very well-regulated system, and normally the size of the rise in your blood sugar and amount of insulin released are in proportion to the foods you eat. If you are sugar sensitive, you can be highly sensitive to car-

bohydrates and your system will overreact. When you eat
carbohydrates, your blood sugar rises more quickly and
goes higher than normal. In response, a greater amount
of insulin is released, and your cells quickly absorb the
sugar in your blood. This causes your blood sugar level to
plunge. These blood sugar changes make you feel really
good, even high, at first, and then tired, overwhelmed,
and spacey as the level drops.

So when a sugar sensitive child eats carbohydrates (especially without protein to slow down the effect), he experiences a blood sugar spike. Instead of a gentle rise and
fall, he gets a spike that causes a problem. This condition
is not the same as hypoglycemia. In hypoglycemia, the
blood sugar drops *below* normal. In sugar sensitivity, the
blood sugar rises and falls quickly but does not necessar-
ily fall below normal. Your sugar sensitive child will run
out of fuel more quickly than other children. If he has
sugary cereal for breakfast at 7 A.M., he will be zooming
around full of energy at 8 and crashing by 9:30. By 10, he
will be both frantic and bouncing off the wall or will be a
zombie, unable to pay attention in class. His body has already used up the sugary cereal, and he's running on
empty. To his teacher, he will look like a child with ADD
or he may seem depressed. It is tricky to diagnose because
the same syndrome can cause different symptoms.

When he is at home and his blood sugar plunges, he
will come cruising into the kitchen for a snack—a sweet
snack NOW! He will drink a soda and grab a Pop-Tart or
a sugar-laden energy bar or grab some candy and dash
out the door. After he eats his snack, his blood sugar will
spike and crash again. This pattern of spiking and crashing
may happen three or four times a day. Each time it does,

it creates stress in your child's body. Each time the blood sugar spikes, the body thinks it is in danger and releases adrenaline. This repeated stress depletes his system more and more. Over time this pattern takes its toll with something called adrenaline fatigue. He crashes on the weekend and sleeps till 9 or 10. During the week, he can't get up on time for school. If you even look at him the wrong way in the morning, he falls apart. He has no resilience. You may attribute his behavior to a growth spurt, or a family issue like a divorce, a move, or the arrival of a new baby. And you wouldn't think to make the connection between this behavior and the sugary cereal he had for breakfast.

Serotonin

Serotonin is a chemical that quiets the brain. It takes the edge off. It makes your child feel like the world is an okay place to be. It also enables her to put the brakes on emotions and behavior. Think of it as the brakes in her brain. If she has a sufficient level of serotonin in her brain, she stays out of trouble. If she doesn't, she can be impulsive, act without thinking, and talk without stopping. A child with low serotonin has a short fuse and talks back. She gets in your face, acts out, and can't control herself. She can get fixed on one subject, one issue, or one desire, and can't get off it. Or she can be depressed, overwhelmed, and unable to cope with stress.

Sugar sensitive children have lower levels of serotonin than other children. Sugar sensitive children who experience trauma or violence (even the violence of movies or video games) will have even lower serotonin and be more vulnerable to the symptoms I have described.

We can't measure exact serotonin levels in the brain, but once you understand the effects of low serotonin, you will begin to see patterns in your child's behavior. If she often manifests the behavior I have described, isn't it a whole lot more comforting to know it is because of imbalanced brain chemistry rather than her just being a bad girl? Or your being a bad parent? Isn't it a relief to know there is a solution that doesn't require expensive medication, psychotherapy, or boot camp? The plan in *Little Sugar Addicts* is designed to raise your child's serotonin levels by making changes in her diet.

Beta-Endorphin

The second brain chemical involved in sugar sensitivity is beta-endorphin. Beta-endorphin is the brain's own pain-killer. It is there to protect us from big pain. When our ancestors had to run from a saber-toothed tiger, their brains flooded with beta-endorphin, which enabled them to keep running despite the pain in their lungs so they could get to safety. In modern times, most people experience that flood of beta-endorphin as a rush called runner's high.

Children who are not sugar sensitive have normal levels of beta-endorphin. They have tolerance for pain; they brush it off with a shake. But sugar sensitive children, who have low beta-endorphin, feel every hurt. They fear or hate the dentist, they cry when they scrape their knees, they cry if they find a dead bird, they cry if a friend hurts their feelings, they cry if you criticize them or even if you look at them the wrong way, they cry at everything, it seems. They are often labeled "sensitive" if they are girls or "sissies" if they are boys.

We have known about the pain-masking effect of beta-endorphin for a long time. But there is a second part of the beta-endorphin story that is even more amazing.

Beta-endorphin levels are also associated with self-esteem. I learned this intriguing fact when I was reading the literature about heroin addicts. Since then, in my work with thousands and thousands of addicts and sugar sensitive people, I have become convinced that this is a crucial part of the story for all of us.

Children with high levels of beta-endorphin feel confident and able to cope with life. When they face hard things, they problem-solve and find solutions. Children with low beta-endorphin get stuck and feel helpless. They feel inadequate and unworthy, even if they are smart. Their feelings do not match the facts. Some of these children overcompensate in an effort to please. They try to be perfect. Others simply give up.

Until I discovered this link, I never imagined that self-esteem was biochemical. Like everyone else, I figured it was psychological. When I raised my own children, I was troubled that they often felt so inadequate. They were attractive, smart, and capable, but the reality didn't seem to matter. What was even more confusing was how their feelings could change. Sometimes they felt they could take on the world, other times they felt like they couldn't even tie their shoes. I often wondered what had I done wrong. It never, ever occurred to me that going for ice cream sundaes was *biochemically* causing their self-esteem to skyrocket right after the sundae and plummet a few hours later.

I first noticed this link between food and self-esteem in my own life. When I was growing up, I often felt the same way my children had. The inside feeling of inadequacy did not match the outside circumstances. There seemed to be no real reason I should feel so unworthy.

After I changed the way I ate, my own self-esteem changed. How I felt on the inside matched the outside. I felt capable, and I was capable. And this feeling didn't suddenly go away one day only to reappear the next. I could count on it. I could count on *myself*.

My experience has now been mirrored in thousands of people who are talking online. Here is a note from Joanne who made a list of her "sugar feelings." Joanne is an adult and was able to articulate the profile pretty clearly. You will see these things in your sugar sensitive children even if they don't have words for them.

- *feeling inadequate*
- *having low self-esteem*
- *feeling victimized*
- *taking things personally*
- *feeling that life is out of control*
- *feeling overwhelmed*
- *overreacting to criticism*
- *living in a "twilight zone"*

There is not a sugar feeling listed here that I have not experienced. I no longer feel any of these feelings on a regular basis. I'm not saying that I no longer ever have a sugar feeling because I do when my food is off. So those are some of the "bad" feelings that I tried to live with before becoming steady on this program. How about the flip side?

- *feeling confident*
- *loving oneself*
- *thinking responsively and reflectively*

- *being other-centered*
- *feeling mobilized and able to take action*
- *thinking clearly and being able to focus*
- *having hope*
- *feeling empowered*
- *staying on an even keel emotionally*

Joanne has captured the essence of the change in beta-endorphin. We called untreated low beta-endorphin the "sugar feelings" phase. When I learned about the relationship of beta-endorphin to self-esteem, I was floored. I often tell the story of working on my Ph.D. research, sitting in the library, and reading a huge text on substance abuse. It must have weighed 20 pounds, and I was squinting to read the tiny text. When I came to a section that talked about the effect of heroin (a beta-endorphin drug) on self-esteem, the hair on the back of my neck stood up. Literally. The text talked about heroin withdrawal and stated that there continued to be "feelings of decreased self-esteem up to 6 months after going off the drug." The implications of this sentence to me were tremendous. I had already learned that sugar activates beta-endorphin, just as heroin does. I made the connection between sugar and self-esteem. The text was suggesting that low self-esteem was a function of withdrawal. My own clinical experience told me that low self-esteem precedes drug use and is one of the primary factors in drug-seeking behavior. Reading that sentence was one of those moments I will remember forever. It literally changed the course of my life.

Sugar and the Link to Addiction

Here's why this discovery was life changing for me, and why it has been life changing for thousands of other sugar sensitive people. Sugar sensitive people are born with low beta-endorphin. Low beta-endorphin produces low self-esteem. It causes you to seek things that raise your beta-endorphin so you feel better about yourself. The substances and experiences that do this quickest tend to be addictive. They include drugs like alcohol, heroin, morphine, and codeine and behaviors like gambling and debting. You remember the rush and go back for more. But after a while you no longer get a rush, and you feel terrible when withdrawal hits. Life becomes a search for ways to stave off the withdrawal. This is the cycle of addiction.

While not deadly like heroin, sugar similarly affects beta-endorphin. It impacts the same neurochemical system as heroin, though not as intensely. Opioid drugs are painkillers that cause their effect by activating beta-endorphin. Heroin, morphine, codeine, Percodan, and Oxy-Contin are all opioid drugs. Sugar acts like an opioid drug in your child's brain. A child with low beta-endorphin will naturally go for what makes her feel better: sugar. And if she has very low levels of beta-endorphin, she will seek her "fix" even more. When you joke about your child being hooked on a can of soda, you are very close to the truth. And when the drug effect wears off, your child will be in opioid withdrawal.

I know it is more than refusal with my son. He gets upset and annoyed when I say no to him. But his reaction is so intense when I cut off his sugar supply. Two cookies with lunch turn into desperate pleas for more cookies or a Popsicle or the dreaded lollipop. The way sugar pacifies him is actually quite disturbing to me.

Marnie

I recently went on a special trip with one of my grandchildren who is sugar sensitive. We were at a wonderful museum of natural history with exhibits of live animals packed with fascinating things to discover. Then she saw an ice cream cone symbol on a sign with an arrow pointing toward the snack bar. ICE CREAM!!! For the next hour the only thing she said was "When will we get ice cream?" No birds, no mountain lions, no prairie dogs, no lunch, no water. Ice cream, and ice cream only, was on her mind. And as soon as she had it (no, I do not tell my children how to raise their children), she was relaxed, funny, cute, charming, and agreeable. Then she fell asleep in the car. My grandchild is three. Think about what happens when your child is six or nine and these patterns are fully established. These are the children who spend all of their allowance on candy and other sweets. These are the children who demand Coke at fast-food restaurants. These are the children who whine, cry, and melt down at Disney World when you have spent $2,000 for a special vacation.

I think I discovered my son was sugar sensitive a few months ago, when he had his first lollipop. I have no doubt that he would eat a dozen of them if I let him. And as soon as you cut him off, he goes into a fit. He was normally such a happy, even-tempered child. He reacts quite strongly to sugar. . . . If I refuse to give him one [lollipop], I have to turn around and leave because he is so irate. But hand him a piece of candy, and it is like someone flipped a switch and he is happy again."

Marnie

What happens to a sugar sensitive child when he turns thirteen and goes into the agony of what we have always assumed to be the natural behavior of early adolescence? Either nothing is right and the world is hopeless, or the world is his oyster, full of possibility and promise. Maybe these highs and lows are simply a function of when he had his last sugar hit and how much soda he had. When you add the effect of beta-endorphin withdrawal to the wide hormonal fluctuations your child is experiencing, adolescence can be hell.

Your child can have an imbalance in any one of these three legs of the sugar sensitive stool or in all three of them. As you come to understand sugar sensitivity, you will start noticing the signs and behaviors of unbalanced brain and body chemistry in your child. You will connect the dots and see that what you thought were separate issues are actually manifestations of the *same* biochemical problem. What you assumed was natural and inevitable is not. You will discover patterns, see where the behavior is coming from, and most important, learn solutions to change it. The key advantage of my treatment for sugar sensitivity is that it goes beyond treating an individual leg and deals with the root cause of the leg imbalances. Treating only one leg keeps things unbalanced. If you give your child Prozac, it deals only with the serotonin piece, not the blood sugar and beta-endorphin pieces. Using food, you can treat and balance all three, at no cost, without drugs or medical intervention, and with no side effects. The food goes to the heart of the issue and balances your child, naturally, gently, safely, and dramatically.

Most important, your children's behavior is not a function of bad parenting. It is not your fault. It is not even their fault. I am not suggesting that you or they have no responsibility for their behavior, but I am suggesting it is driven by the biochemistry. Once you grasp the power of sugar sensitive biochemistry, you will no longer carry the burden of not understanding why your children act the way they do. Even more significantly, once you understand how diet affects your child's biochemistry, you will be empowered to make changes that heal the problem.

Little Sugar Addicts will give you a road map for making these changes. It will show you how food can heal your child *and* your family. It will provide a specific series of "baby steps" that your family will not only accept but actually buy in to and truly believe in. The guidelines will help you help your family to establish new eating patterns and new behaviors, as thousands of families have already done.

You are not alone with this issue. We will work the solution together. You will have support, and the results will seem miraculous. Healing sugar sensitivity will transform how you feel about your life, how your children feel about their lives, and how you feel about each other.

2

It Is Not Your Fault,
There Is a Solution

I am convinced that the biochemistry of sugar sensitivity is an underlying factor in alcoholism, addiction, depression, ADD, obesity, and diabetes. A diet high in sugars and refined carbohydrates, low in quality protein, high in saturated fat, and low in essential fatty acids, eaten in erratic and poorly timed meals, creates behavioral havoc and sets up huge emotional and physical problems in the future.

As diets get more and more compromised, these problems are showing up in younger and younger children. Junk foods, soda in the schools, and missed meals activate the worst of what sugar sensitivity sets up. As a parent, you may not make this connection between food and behavior until you get some sort of wake-up call. The day a school guidance counselor suggests your child take Ritalin smacks you in the face more harshly than a headline about the rising incidence of ADD. Perhaps you have made the painful trek to pediatricians, psychologists, and counselors. But rarely does anyone talk to you about nutrition. In fact, I bet when you have raised diet as a factor, you were dismissed as grasping at straws and handed a prescription for a drug.

But the fact is, your intuition is right on. The science underlying my theory of sugar sensitivity is solid, well researched, and presented in serious medical journals. Elliott Blass talks about the drug effect of sugar, Christine Gianoulakis has clearly shown that low beta-endorphin is passed down in alcoholic families, and recently Bart Hoebel has replicated sugar addiction in rats. If you want the in-depth science, check the Bibliography at the end of this book. Or get *Potatoes Not Prozac* and read the science chapter. And perhaps more significantly, the lived experience of thousands of parents like you can guide you into trusting that hunch, acting on it, and making changes in your family. Sugar sensitivity is real, and you can heal it by changing what and when you eat.

Now that you have a sense that your children may be sugar sensitive, let's begin the task of making some change. It is very easy to jump to the idea of simply changing your kids' food and having their behavior shape right up. That is exactly what I do *not* want you to do. Forced change right off the bat will not work. We have some thinking and some homework to do first. Having your children buy into making change will mean that the process will stick over time. It won't be just one more crazy thing mom wants to try. We are looking for long-term, systematic, and lasting change. It is crucial for the kids to participate. I say, don't do this *for* your children, do it *with* your children. Creating a *buy-in*, albeit sometimes reluctantly, is the single biggest factor in making a successful transition in the family food.

But how to get a buy-in? Those little addicts are not

about to give up their sugar! This may shock you, but you start the process with yourself. Children learn from imitating their parents. Much as you would like to believe that isn't true, the single biggest factor in the healing equation is *your* behavior. You need to do what you are asking them to do. The lived experience of watching Mom or Dad make the changes is the single biggest motivator you can give them. Your children remember the mood swings, the unpredictability, the fatigue, the forgetting or not keeping promises that were part of mom's active "sugar days." They may never talk about it with you, but they know. And they notice when you are relaxed and funny. They notice no more yelling, no more inconsistency. They love doing fun things with you.

Their little brains do register the connection between food and mood.

I had an incident last night that made me chuckle. My son (8) came in crying and obviously afraid to tell me something. He finally told me that he had put a gash in the wall in the front room, the one I just repainted. I had told everyone to be careful in there and to try not to mark up the walls.

I think he was amazed when I told him not to worry about it and just try to be more careful in the future. I think he expected to be in real trouble. I guess he isn't used to the new and improved "no yelling" me. A few months ago the mar on the wall would have upset me, now I just shrug it off and am able to chuckle at his reaction to me.

Ain't life grand when you are radiant.

Vicki

When you picked this book up, you may have felt that it was going to be about fixing your kids. You may not have made the connection to the idea that sugar sensitivity is a family story. You are part of it. Whether your family is Mom and Dad and kids or Mom and partner and kids, or Grandma and kids, or Dad and kids, it doesn't matter. Healing sugar sensitivity is a family affair. *You* have to buy in first; *you* have to buy in for yourself. This plan will not work if you think you can just fix them and not yourself.

You Are Part of the Solution

Sugar sensitive kids are the smartest, most intuitive folks in the world. Don't try to fool them. They will catch you in the act. Flat out, they will know how silly the idea of "do what I say, not what I do" is. When you are in a sugar fog, you forget the power of their knowing. You think you can get away with doing something different from what you are asking your children to do. The reality is your children know. They notice every little nuance of how you are. Bottom line? You have to start your own program first. There is no fudging, so to speak, on this one.

You don't have to be completely fixed before you get your kids started. That could be a long wait. You just have to start first. Why? Because I want you relaxed and focused in planning family change. I want your own biochemistry to be an ally rather than an enemy in the process. Making change with your children will take some commitment. If you start from your own strength and healing, things will work better. If you are tired and cranky and in sugar withdrawal and they start in, you will cave pretty quickly. You will be at the head of the line for

Dairy Queen. You will be thrilled to make cookies for school so you can eat the dough. You can't fix your kids unless you are steady.

I have not started this because I find the thought of trying to do this with two children who are every bit as addicted to sugar as I am ABSOLUTELY DAUNTING. In the past when I have tried to keep sugar out of the house, not only have they stolen money to buy candy and ice cream at school, but I'd have to listen to their constant whining. It drove me nuts, and so I gave up.

Gracie

If you start with the basics, keep things simple, and put your own oxygen mask on first, the plan will work for all of you.

Thank you so much for the encouragement! After really looking at my [food] journal yesterday (only my second day) I noticed a major thing. After I eat sugar, I get really perky and social. I stay that way for about three hours. Then when it wears off, I am the most grouchy person you've ever met! And the littlest things set me off. I always thought I needed to work on not being such a grouch, when for once, now I know I am not to blame. It's the sugar! I can't wait to be normal again!

Amanda

Actually, it will work beyond anything in your wildest dreams. It will literally change your entire family's way of being in the world. And most important, it will change the course of your child's life. You will be doing something that really matters. But you have to go slowly, you have to do baby steps, and you have to start with yourself first.

> *"I had absolutely no patience with [my kids] and no energy to do anything but what had to be done. We almost never had any fun together. This program has meant a world of difference to [my son] Mike and my relationship with him as well as my other children. Not only am I more stable, but Mike doesn't have headaches anymore, and he is a much sweeter, easy-to-deal-with child. I'm truly enjoying my children for the first time ever. He even reads labels now to see if there's sugar in the drinks that he's offered!*
>
> *Katy*

As you start to think about your own process, let me take you back to the intriguing idea I introduced in the previous chapter—the connection between sugar sensitivity, low beta-endorphin, and low self-esteem. Think about how that information touched you and how the idea of your child's sense of self is powered by biochemistry. This same process drives you. It isn't just your child we are dealing with. If you have not yet balanced your own sugar sensitive chemistry, you can feel the same way. You may be skilled and competent but feel inadequate and unable to cope. If *you* are off balance, dealing with your child's behavior will be extremely difficult. When you are off balance, it is very hard to cope with anything more than just getting by. The idea of getting your family healthy will sound great, but the practical reality can be daunting.

If you are sugar sensitive and your own food is off, changing your family's food will not work. You will be excited by the ideas, but things will not change. This will be just one more flash in the pan. What is at stake is too important. So we start with the key player: you.

> *In recent months I have shifted my primary focus from my children to MYSELF. It has made a huge difference in my life. I am feeling better about myself now more than ever. I'm more laid back, I play more, I laugh more, I rest more. Through it all, I've discovered that I'm being the best role model I can for my children.*
>
> *Gail*

If you are not convinced that you are a part of the equation, let's take a little sidetrack and see if you are sugar sensitive. Take the chocolate chip cookie test, my favorite old standby. Imagine that you are alone. You come home and someone has been baking in your house. There is a plate of warm chocolate chip cookies on the counter. What kind of reaction would you have? Do your molecules light up at even the idea of warm chocolate chip cookies? Or perhaps warm scones? Or ice cream? Perhaps you would not actually eat them, but the crucial part is the wanting to. People who are not sugar sensitive would not care about the cookies.

Does this sound like you? A sugar sensitive child will have a sugar sensitive parent or grandparent. If the chocolate chip cookie test does not resonate with you, you may not be sugar sensitive. If that is the case, you won't need to make changes for yourself, specifically. If you are not sugar sensitive but your child is, it is likely that your child's other parent is. Keep reading and see what you think.

Passing the chocolate chip cookie test does not mean you are bad. Remember, this is about biochemistry and diet, not personality, parenting skills, or moral fiber! And the good news is, we have a way to address the biochemistry through diet. How? Through the seven very straightforward steps that are the basis of my three previous books, *Potatoes Not Prozac*, *The Sugar Addict's Total Recovery Program*, and *Your Last Diet!* I won't be going into those seven steps in detail here—you can consult the books if you want more information—but the first two steps will help you get started in creating the safety net for your child. Here they are:

- Have breakfast with the *right amount of protein and complex carbohydrates* every morning within an hour of waking up.
- Keep a journal that tracks the relationship between what you are eating and how you are feeling.

At first glance these two steps may appear to be incredibly simple. Breakfast, food journal. Oftentimes sugar sensitive folks, impulsive as they are, will say, "Right! Got it!" and whip right through both steps in three days. Nope, not what we want here. Start at the beginning. Go slowly. First spend time with breakfast.

Breakfast, Protein, and You

First of all, calculate how much protein you will need by taking one half your body weight and using that for your daily protein needs in grams. For instance, you weigh 150 pounds you will need around 75 grams of protein per day, or 25 grams per meal.

This is probably more protein than you are currently eating. If your breakfast is along the lines of coffee and yogurt, you will need to find ways to add protein. An 8-ounce container of yogurt contains only 8 grams of protein, and coffee has none. Many of us make a protein shake for breakfast. This tradition started at my treatment clinic as some of the guys found it impossible to cope with breakfast. My senior counselor, George, helped me develop a tasty mix of protein and complex carbohydrates. The clients referred to it as "George's Shake" and a tradition started. Since the publication of *Potatoes Not Prozac* thousands and thousands of us have made a habit of drinking George's Shake on the way to work. You can either make a variation of it yourself by using the recipe on page 67 or the variations in the back of the book (see page 212) or you can order a mix directly from our website at www.radiantrecovery.com.

Below are some other quick and easy breakfast ideas. They are simply to give you a sense of the kinds of foods our community are having for their first meal. You will need to adjust the protein amounts to suit your weight. You will see that each breakfast combines some protein food and carbohydrate food. This is not a diet, this is about healing. Do not worry about having whole grains or taking out the sugar yet. The key here is having enough protein, combined with some carbohydrates, and having it within an hour of getting up.

- scrambled eggs, sausage, and toast
- George's Shake made with oat milk
- pancakes or waffles made with protein powder in the batter, with applesauce and yogurt
- ham, cheese, and broccoli omelet with hash browns

- beef or chicken with bean burrito
- oatmeal with protein powder, milk or yogurt, and fruit
- two hard-boiled eggs, toast, and an orange to have in the car on the way to work
- bagel with lox and cream cheese piled high
- cottage cheese mixed with fresh fruit, and a muffin
- corned beef hash and two eggs with a slice of toast

Even if you are not able to get the protein you need right away, start with what you can do. Increase your protein and have breakfast every morning even if you are not sugar sensitive. Master what *you* will have before trying to figure out what you will give your children. Start off by being entirely selfish. Find something that is easy and tasty and that you can do. It doesn't matter if you have the same thing seven days a week. Find your breakfast, find your routine, and you will be amazed at what a difference just this one thing does. Remember to have it within an hour of waking up. Your blood sugar has dropped during the night. You are running on empty. It is easy to forget to eat. Your hunger mechanism probably doesn't work well. Train yourself for breakfast—breakfast with protein— every morning.

Keeping a Food Journal

After you have mastered breakfast, and grown to love it, start a food journal. The journal is not a diet log. It is a way for your body to talk with you. It allows your body to be your partner in the process. Your body will guide you by giving you symptoms. Fatigue, headaches, irritability, relaxation, and focus are all clues. Your journal will help you make connections between what and when you eat and how you feel.

You can use any notebook for your journal or you can purchase the one we designed called *Your Body Speaks*, available through bookstores or our website (www. radiantrecovery.com). You will want to record what and when you eat, how much you have, how you feel physically, and how you feel emotionally. Make a column for each section so that you can easily make connections. Here is what each journal page will look like:

Date and Time	What You Eat or Drink	How You Feel Physically	How You Feel Emotionally

Write in your journal whenever you eat or drink something. Record your feelings as you experience them, not just at mealtimes. If you do not want to carry the journal around with you, jot notes and then fill it out when you get home. At first, it will be hard to remember to write in your journal. Life will intrude, you will forget, you will misplace your journal. Or you may not want to look at how you eat. You may think, "How silly is this! I want to help my kids!" Be patient and do the best you can. Think of your journal as your body's voice. It wants to help you help it to feel better. Once you notice that, yes, you crash every day at three P.M., you will start having more control over how you feel.

I have written lots and lots about journaling in my other books, *Potatoes Not Prozac, The Sugar Addict's Total Recovery Program,* and *Your Last Diet!* If you get stuck, check out the recommendations in any of those books. We also have an entire e-mail support list called Radiant Journal on our website at www.radiantrecovery.com. You can click on the link that says Online Support Groups to join. Work with your journal for a few weeks, and it will get easier over time. After you have been doing the journal for a while, you will be ready to start with your kids.

Tracking Your Family's Eating Habits

I think I have to treat his addiction the same way I am treating mine. If I do it too fast, I'm setting him up for pain and failure. I got his little body into this, and I want to make sure I do it in the safest, most effective way possible.

Marnie

I know you want to get on with changing your family's diet right now. Bear with me. Before you start making changes, I want you to simply get a sense of what you are really dealing with in your children's diets. Your job right now is very, very simple. You will make no changes. You are simply going to pay attention and start learning what and when your children eat. This task is a real eye-opener. It is important that you come to it with a sense of objectivity. Don't judge yourself as a parent, and don't be horrified by what your children are eating. Simply get some information.

For one week, I want you to notice and write down what you observe. Use a different notebook from the one you are using for yourself. For the first week, do not tell your children you are doing this exploration. Make it your private detective work. Do one child at a time if you have more than one at home. Notice what you can without asking too many questions. If your children get lunch at school, assume they eat what is served. Do not probe, do not explore, just get the school lunch menu. If the school uses fast-food vendors, ask your kids what they usually get. Don't make a big deal of it. Think of yourself as the stealth recorder. It will be important to guesstimate portion sizes as well as you can. Is your child eating a half-cup of Cheerios or a full cup? How much milk really went into the bowl?

If you are a working mom, you may not be entirely aware of everything your children eat during the day, especially when they are not in school. See if you can gather some clues by observing changes in the cupboard. What do you have in the house for snacks? How has it changed over the week? Do you start on Monday with three liters of soda that are gone by Friday? As you deepen your detective work, evaluate the crime scene.

And now add another piece to the puzzle. After you get home from a trip to the grocery store, check off your groceries as you unpack them against the cash register receipt. I want you to be ultra-aware of what you buy in a typical week. Here is the method. Start by making a list— the cash register receipt will do. Take the list and look at it. Make some notes. Categorize what you bought. What kinds of proteins did you get? How much meat, eggs, fish, or cottage cheese? What vegetables did you get? Make a note of both the type and the amount. What fruits? What bread? What cereals? What snack foods? Count soda, juice, coffee, beer, or whatever other drinks you get for your family.

Get a sense of what proportion of your foods come from the grocery store and what proportion come from eating out. Perhaps you have been to Sam's or Costco and remember how they review your receipt at the door. I want you to do the same thing when you get home. Take the receipt and sit down and go over it. I want you to move from unconscious to conscious. This may be hard. You may not want to know this information. You may have some shame around it. You may not like what you find. Try hard not to judge yourself. Gather facts. You need to know the data in order to plan change.

You may have a household that mostly eats out. If so, you will want to do this exercise a little differently. Perhaps you never really go to the store once a week. Perhaps you and your husband or partner picks things up on the way home from work. If this is your style, then simply pay attention to a week's worth of take-out and occasional groceries. I want you to get a clear sense of what your family eats each week and what each child eats. Do not get overwhelmed or obsessed by this process. You are trying to uncover the big picture, and I want you to have fun.

Now sit down and figure out how much you spend on food for your family for a week. List the amounts you spend at the grocery store, at the convenience store, and on eating out.

What snack foods do you get? Pay really close attention to this. Are you getting little individual things for lunches? Bags of chips for afternoon snacks? Microwave popcorn? What dessert foods? What breakfast foods? How much soda do you get? What kind? Individual or in liter or two-liter bottles?

As you start this process, you may want to cheat and start making changes right away. Resist that urge! Keep going with your detective work first. Much of the fun down the line will come with noticing the change. You won't have the fun of seeing the change unless you know where you started. So keep working at this task. Don't jump ahead even though that is what sugar sensitive people love to do! You may vow to stop buying soda immediately, but unless you take the baby steps outlined in Chapter 3, you will be setting yourself and your family up for failure. You need a foundation in place first. If you don't get the buy-in, you will just create a need to go around the program, to sabotage your efforts, and sneak sweets. This is exactly what you do *not* want to do. Be patient, and go slowly. Let's make it work long term.

Now that you have a general sense of the lay of the land, let's take it to another level. Remember, you are simply gathering the data. No analysis yet. Once you have the preliminary info, talk to your kids about what you are doing. Frame it as a crime-scene investigation. Share with them that you are learning about how diet affects behavior. Make this fun so they don't get spooked. Have your kids help you fill in the gaps for what they eat. Make a set of big charts. One for each child. Have them help you fill in the blanks. Ask them what they had for lunch, for snacks. Be funny or they will lie. Make it a game. Use different color markers. Get some pads of large paper. I like the giant-sized adhesive Post-it notes that will stick to the wall. Use one sheet for each member of the family.

Start with a day, and then do a week. How are your kids different from one another? See if you can distinguish some patterns. Anthony always has food with him and grazes throughout the day. Marie skips breakfast, hates lunch, and eats all evening. Daddy forgets breakfast and eats lunch out at a restaurant every day. Have the kids help tease out these small details and patterns. Approach it as a crime-scene investigation and be interested in every tiny detail.

Now it may be that your kids make it a point not to tell you what they really eat. They may not want you to know that they had soda and chips for lunch. They certainly don't want to tell you that they tossed the lunch you made them, or that they used their lunch money for candy. Gently remember that little addicts hide their truth. Many of us did as children, so it is not at all unusual to think that your kids might do the same. If you are funny about this, they are more likely to be honest. If they resist, simply leave their page blank. Blank gives you information. Don't skip a beat, work with the kids who want to share.

Using the Data

If you can get your kids excited, they may decide to share in this exploration. Now that you have some data to work with, change will be fun. See if you can figure out three things:

- how much protein your children eat each day
- the level of their junk food consumption
- how much sugar they eat

To start, you will need to invest in a pocket nutrition reference book that lists the protein grams of many foods. You can find this kind of book in the diet section of any bookstore or even at the grocery store, or you can go on-line for the information. There are a number of nutrition software programs that provide this information; I like LifeForms at www.fitnesoft.com. Better yet, send your kids online. The more they participate in this exercise, the more meaning it will have for them. Remember, just gather information, and don't comment on it. Have your kids count the total grams of protein they have in a day. Let them calculate this for an entire week, and then calculate their average daily protein intake. Even if they are little, these exercises will be fun.

Your next step is to identify the junk food you all eat. Don't scare the kids by being judgmental about it. Tell them you want to see if they all eat the same kinds of things or if they have different tastes. Do you have a potato chip eater or a candy eater or both? Give each child a three-by-five index card to record the junk food they eat for a week. Before you start, sit everyone down together to decide what junk food means in your house. Sort out the difference between fast food and junk food. Each family will define it a little differently. If your children are little, you can make up a food card with pictures for them. They can check off what they eat during the week. Have them tailor their card to the foods and places in their world. For example, you can draw an M for McDonald's, a crown for Burger King, and a bell for Taco Bell. Identify the choices together. Make it fun. Remember, no judgment. You are doing fact-finding. The purpose of doing the junk foods separately is to get a profile of what your junk-food junkies are drawn to. The overall food profile will show up on the sheets you all do together. The junk-food part is a refinement of that exercise to identify the "drugs" of choice of each family member. You need to participate in this and be humorous about your own favorite things. If you have another adult in the house, make sure to include him or her. Let your kids tease you about the special need for junk food you might have. It will help them connect to their own special things.

Now this may seem like a huge amount of extra work for you. Why in heaven's name are we bothering with all of this? Why not just get these kids off sugar? A good part of addiction is denial and unconscious behavior. We are starting a process of waking up. We want to do it slowly. If you take your time, include your children, and try to make this process creative and fun, you will be building a strong foundation for change. They will have a better sense of what you are talking about when the time comes to cut certain foods out. And if you know what you are really dealing with, you will be able to make informed choices about which things to take out first. This exercise will give you a way to meet each child where she or he is. If you discover that Billy has an inordinate attachment to Ding Dongs, you can ease into that arena slowly. Or if you discover that you buy five boxes of Pop-Tarts a week, you know what your family is attached to for breakfast. This clue will teach you that you won't ditch them right off the bat.

Looking at the Sugars

Now let's add the third scan of our detective program. Let's look at how much sugar your family eats. This one is a little trickier than figuring out grams of protein. Most of the foods your children eat will have a sugar content listed on the nutritional information label, as part of the carbohydrate content. This number is not an accurate measure of the real sugar content. It is measuring only the sugars that are legally classified as such, like sucrose. Sugars such as dextrose are legally classified as complex carbohydrates, so they are included in the total carbohydrate count but not in the sugar content. For this exercise, have your kids do two things. Count the actual carbohydrate grams, and then list the sugars in the foods they eat each day. Here is a list of sugars, in alphabetical order. It may not be complete since manufacturers generate new sugars all the time.

barley malt	galactose	molasses
beet sugar	glucose	polydextrose
brown rice syrup	granulated sugar	powdered sugar
brown sugar	high fructose corn syrup	raisin juice
cane juice	honey	raisin syrup
confectioners' sugar	invert sugar	raw sugar
corn sweetener	lactose	sorbitol
corn syrup	maltodextrin	SUCANAT
date sugar	malted barley	sucrose
dextrin	maltitol	sugar cane
dextrose	maltose	turbinado sugar
fructooliosaccharides	mannitol	white sugar
fructose	maple sugar	xylitol
fruit juice concentrate	microcrystalline cellulose	

Have your kids copy this list onto an index card. Encourage ruthless detective skills. When you go for fast foods, have them look at the label on the packet of mayonnaise to find high fructose corn syrup and corn syrup solids. You don't need to comment, just encourage them. Make it a contest to see how many of these sugars they can find and check off on their cards. Give a prize to the child who discovers the most sugar names. See if anyone finds a new sugar. (The prize should not be a sweet.) Make this fun. We want to take the negative charge off the process of "waking up" and stepping out of denial.

As you are doing these exercises with your children, make sure you do them as well. Record what you eat. Be open about your list. Model fact-finding. The more you are able to do this, the more you will help everyone get out of unconscious eating or shame and hiding. Make jokes about being the Sugar Queen (if you are). Talk about the King of Coke, the Prince of Ice Cream. You want to shift all the negative messages that you and your children have been hearing about how bad all these things are. By taking the negative charge off, you are starting the process of moving your family out of denial and into the great buy-in. Humor heals.

After you have spent some time gathering all this information, you will be ready to put it together to get a sense of where your kids are. What are they eating? What levels of protein are they having each day? Don't try to calculate how much protein they need at this point. The formula for children is a little different from the one I gave you to work out your own protein needs. I want you to just stick with fact-finding for now. I will talk about how to calculate their protein needs in Chapter 3.

What kinds of protein do they eat? Are they picky eaters, or are they willing to eat anything? How much sugar are they having? What kinds of sweets are they drawn to? Do they love hard-core sugars, or are they mostly drawn to breads and cereals?

After you have reviewed your data, I want you to hold a family debriefing. Gather all the kids together, and share what you have learned. Ask them if your assessment of their food seems on target. Ask for their opinion. Ask them to refine and critique your assessment. Remember, it is absolutely critical that you remain nonjudgmental throughout this process. You may be thinking, "Dear heavens, Billy is drinking three Cokes a day, eating chips for lunch, and picking at dinner." Yep, that may be true. And it *will* change. But not yet. You have to contain your distress and remain a detached observer for this to work.

You are planting the seeds of the great buy-in. As your children start to get a sense of what they eat, you will have a foundation to make change. If you just tell them to stop having sugar, or you just force change, you will simply lay the groundwork for some major eating problems in the future. You are actually starting the process of moving your family out of denial. You are not going to "break" it; you are going to heal it. You are dealing with little bodies that are biochemically dependent upon the effects of sugars. You live with a group of little sugar addicts who have a vested interest in keeping these "drugs." You yourself may be part of the addicted family system. You have started the process of taking the shame off and seeing this as a biochemical problem—a problem that can be resolved. If you can start looking at the equation with an eye to healing the addiction, you will be on the way to making profound change.

The Myth of "Just Say No"

Contrary to what some folks say, "Just say no" does not work with addiction. The people who can successfully just say no are those who have a different biochemistry than you or your children. They do not experience withdrawal, they do not have cravings, they do not have an emotional attachment to what they eat in the same way you do. They are not sugar sensitive. They are the same people who will tell you to "just take your children off of sugar." At best this message is a functional instruction. At worst it carries an implicit condemnation of your parenting skills. That message of "why don't you just . . ." is very pervasive in our culture.

That message is at the root of your shame. If it were that simple, you would have stopped the sugar long ago. I am taking you through a process that will *heal* your addiction, not break it. You will feel safe, understood, and guided throughout the process because I know the biochemistry of addiction so well. I understand what is happening in your children's brains and bodies; I understand what is driving their behaviors. I have no judgments about it. If Tony has a temper tantrum, I do not think he is a spoiled child or you are a bad parent. I know if his blood sugar is crashing, he is having sugar withdrawal. And soon enough, you are going to know all this, too. The frustration and aggravation will fade, and you will start seeing profound changes in your children.

Creating the Solution

By now, I suspect that you know your children are sugar sensitive and you are ready for the solution. Your review of your family's eating habits has pretty much convinced you that change needs to be made. You are ready to do whatever it takes to heal your children.

Surprisingly, the key challenge will be to go *slowly*. If you make too much change too fast, you will create chaos and resentment. You will set yourself and your family up for failure and lose time. You will go backward rather than forward. The healing steps for children are based on the idea of abundance, not deprivation. You are going to *add* good foods in before you take any foods out. You will create biochemical stability before you make change.

If you have been working on your own program, or have read any of my other books, you know that we have seven steps. Now we have developed seven different steps for children. They are not the same as the adult steps because children's bodies are different from adult bodies; children are not just small adults. They have different metabolic needs, and their sugar sensitivity imbalances manifest in a slightly different way.

Let's look at the seven steps for children first. Read them, and then let me walk you through each of them.

1. Eat breakfast with protein.
2. Make connections between food and mood.
3. Change snacks and drinks.
4. Eat protein lunches.
5. Shift to whole grain food.
6. Take out the sugar.
7. Take care of life.

Notice that taking out sugar is not step one. It is step six, not step one. As I have pointed out, before you start taking anything out of your child's diet, you will want to add in some things like protein. You want to balance your child's biochemistry and heal the brain before taking out the sugar. Your enthusiasm may outpace your child's capacity to integrate the change, so we do not want to rush. Remember to think of this as a program of abundance rather than deprivation. Do the steps in order, slowly. Slowly means six to eighteen months to go through them all. Here is why slower is better.

- Going slower puts attention on the process rather than on the end, which most people define as getting off sugar. It allows your child to get to know a given step rather than blazing through.
- Going slower reinforces following instructions. Sugar sensitive people tend not to do this.
- Going slower gives you a chance to learn the drill so you can better lead your children through it.
- Going slower allows the behavioral changes your child is making to settle in. These include planning, stopping, waiting, and not acting impulsively.
- Going slower allows the neurological change to "set" with each step before you make more change.
- Going slower reduces the number of variables your child is dealing with and trying to pay attention to.

3

Step One:
Breakfast with Protein

Breakfast is the foundation of all the steps. Breakfast provides an anchor for your child who has volatile blood sugar and does not do well with long intervals between eating. If your child had dinner at six the night before and got up at seven in the morning, he has gone thirteen hours without food. Imagine going from breakfast to dinner thirteen hours later. It is unthinkable. Yet parents often let breakfast slip. Or they think that a bowl of cereal and milk will do the job. Your child needs more protein than just milk for the brain and more carbohydrates for sustained energy. Step one is pretty straightforward. I call it Breakfast with Protein, but really it has four parts.

- **Regularity:** Make sure you have it every morning.
- **Timing:** Have it within an hour of getting up.
- **Amount:** Have enough protein for your body.
- **Balance:** Have some good carbohydrates with it.

Deciding on a breakfast that includes all of these may take some work. Work on the four parts in order. Up to now breakfast may have been a fly-out-the-door affair. You may have been handing your child a breakfast bar as she dashes to the bus. Or you may be giving him money to pick up something on the way to school. You may simply be giving the younger kids a bowl of cereal while you try to pry the older ones out of bed. You may all leave in a rush, they may leave before you do, and they may bounce out the door without your thinking much of it. Until you did the food journaling outlined in the last chapter, you may not have known what your children are eating. But now, because you took the time to gather the information, you have data.

Not too long ago I taught a class to a group of sixth graders. I asked them to share what they had for breakfast. Here's the list:

Maria	Brownies and Coke
Sally	Cap'n Crunch
Ricki	Bagel with cream cheese and orange juice
Larissa	Kix
Jennifer	Ravioli
Anna Marie	Toast with jelly, coffee with sugar
Susie	Gatorade and chicken nuggets
Alex	Cinnamon roll, oatmeal
Marcia	Biscuits, milk, hot chocolate
Max	Cornflakes
Mitch	Honey Bunches of Oats
Honey	Plain yogurt and fruit and whole grain toast

The survey made a big impact on the teacher. She had attributed the behaviors of the class to hormones. When she heard about their breakfasts, she realized that the impact of diet was huge.

Since then I have done a similar survey several more times. The sixth graders' breakfast choices seem to be a representative starting point for many middle-school children. But they won't do for a sugar sensitive child. They are not enough food, and they do not provide the right nutrients for brain stability. Even Honey's breakfast is light on protein. It is fine if your child is eating this way now. No shame. Think of it as the starting point.

Breakfast: Every Day and On Time

Let's break down the process of having a good breakfast every morning into some baby steps. The first is to always, always have *something* to eat every morning. Children cannot skip breakfast, and they need to eat within an hour of getting up. Your first task is to set a rule that everyone in your house (including you) will have breakfast within an hour of waking up every morning of every day. Tell your family that breakfast needs to include some protein and some sort of complex carbohydrate. You are not being punitive or harsh. You are simply setting a new ground rule of the house. No skipping, and have the right food. Have a family meeting with your kids to let them know you are setting a new ground rule and that you are going to need their help.

Of course, you need to give them some context or they will be totally confused. Why is Mom suddenly doing this breakfast thing? Is this some new fad or what? Talk with them about sugar sensitivity. Show them this book. Share the food and behavior connection. Tell them what you are learning and how much you want their brains to work well. You do not need to provide an entire course in the brain chemistry of sugar sensitivity, but giving them background on this new commitment will help them make the change.

As you start setting new ground rules, you may run smack into a dilemma that will hound you in every step— finding the balance between telling your kids what to do and having them buy in and make healthy choices. Here is the tactic that has worked over and over among our online community parents. You choose certain things that are nonnegotiable, and then you have your children make choices within these parameters. In your heart of hearts, you must be willing to say that breakfast is not negotiable, that it must be eaten within an hour of getting up, and that it has to include some basic things. *They* can choose what kinds of proteins and carbohydrate to have, but you must hold your ground on the basic expectation of having breakfast every morning.

Talk with your children before it is a problem, when they are rested and fed and attentive. Say, "I don't ever want to fight with you on this, but it is really important for all of us. " Find a solution for every concern before the fact. Little sugar addicts who are still using their drug of choice (sugar) are not equipped to make the best choices or have reasonable logic. Don't have unrealistic expectations for little mush-brains. Set the big boundary, and then help them explore the choices on how to do it. You send the message, "Breakfast is not negotiable."

And make sure you are "doing breakfast" with them.

They need to know that you mean it and will do it, too. If you are not convinced and you are mushy, they will know it. They will pick the morning you are late and have to leave on time or when your mother-in-law is visiting to argue. Having the right breakfast within an hour needs to be like wearing a seat belt—you don't argue, you don't let it escalate into a power struggle, you just do it. Your energy on the issue of breakfast will make a huge difference in how they accept the change.

Getting Enough Protein

Most kids love to solve riddles and puzzles and will enjoy figuring out how much protein they need at breakfast. Calculating this for children is a little trickier than for adults. For adults, I suggest 0.5 grams per pound per day. If you weigh 150 pounds, you should have about 75 grams of protein per day or about 25 per meal. But adults are not growing and are not making brain and body cells every day.

The rule of thumb for children is to have between 0.7 and 1.0 grams of protein per pound of their body weight per day until they are eighteen. The total amount will be spaced out between three meals and two snacks. The actual amount will depend on how active your child is and whether he is going through a growth spurt. This does not have to be an exact calculation. It is simply a guideline to make sure your children get enough and not too much. If your child is playing soccer and growing, you must make sure the amount is at the upper end of the scale. A child who sits a lot or who is getting pudgy will be eating at the lower end of the scale. If you have a thirty-pounder who is not growing this month, then she will need 21 grams of protein per day or about 5 grams per meal and 3 grams at each snack. Make sure that the daily total is spread evenly through the day. Don't give her a huge breakfast and a very light lunch. Here is a chart to help you see what this would mean for different-size children. I am using weights rather than ages so you can follow the recommendations more easily.

Child's Weight	Total Grams of Protein in the Day	Grams of Protein in a Meal	Grams of Protein in a Snack
30 pounds	21–30	5–10	2–5
40 pounds	28–40	7–12	3–7
50 pounds	35–50	10–15	5–9
60 pounds	42–60	15–20	7–10
75 pounds	48–75	18–25	10–12
80 pounds	55–80	20–25	10–12

Now, don't let these numbers make you crazy. These are simply a rough guide to estimate a good amount for your child. Learn how much protein is in certain foods, and see what this means in terms of portion size. For a small child weighing 40 pounds, it means that one egg for breakfast and a cheese stick as a snack are perfect. Most parents are surprised by how little a small child needs and how much a sixth grader playing sports needs. The key is to listen to your child and see how the behavior changes. When the amount of food is on target, you will know by how your child acts.

Start the calculation process *with* your children. Make it a game, especially for kids who like numbers and problem solving. Once you and your child have determined how much protein in grams they need at each meal based on weight and activity, you will be ready to figure out how much food to serve. First, let's identify some protein foods that work for most children:

Dairy [milk, cheese, yogurt]
Eggs
Fish [tuna, salmon, white fish, trout]
Poultry [chicken, turkey]
Meat [beef, pork]
Beans and nuts

Sit down with your children and help them identify the proteins they like. Some families with young children make a scrapbook with pictures of proteins. Others cut out pictures from magazines and put them up on the refrigerator. Calculating the amount of grams in each type of food is a little tricky but doable.

Dense protein sources (meat, chicken, fish) contain more grams of protein per ounce than not-so-dense sources (legumes, nuts, cheese). Meat, poultry, and fish have somewhere between 7 and 9 grams of protein in each ounce. So, for example, a 3-ounce chicken breast has 21–27 grams of protein. Eggs have 7–9 grams of protein per egg depending on the size. Beans have 8–9 grams of protein in a half-cup cooked serving.

The chart on page 60 will give you a sense of the relative protein grams in foods you might typically use, as well as children's need for protein.

Food	Amount	Grams of Protein	30-Pound Child (8 grams average recommended amount per meal)	40-Pound Child (10 grams average recommended amount per meal)	60-Pound Child (16 grams average recommended amount per meal)
Egg	1 large	7	1	1.5	2
Peanut butter	2 Tbsp.	7	2 Tbsp.	2½ Tbsp.	4 Tbsp. (¼ c.)
Bologna	1 slice	2.8	3 slices	3½ slices	6 slices
Hot dog	1	8	1	1½	2
Sliced ham	1 slice	4	2 slices	2½ slices	4 slices
Yogurt	8 oz.	16	4 oz.	5 oz.	8 oz.
Milk	8 oz.	8	1 c.	10 oz.	2 c.
Seeds like sunflower and pumpkin	1 oz.	7	1 oz.	1½ oz.	2 oz.
Cottage cheese	4 oz.	14	2 oz.	3 oz.	4 oz.
Cheese	1 oz.	5	1½ oz.	2 oz.	4 oz.
Whey protein powder	1 scoop	16	½ scoop	¾ scoop	1 scoop
Hamburger	1 oz.	8	1 oz.	1½ oz.	2 oz.
Chicken	1 oz.	8	1 oz.	1½ oz.	2 oz.
Tuna	1 oz.	8	1 oz.	1½ oz.	2 oz.

As you look at this chart, you may have questions like "What brand of peanut butter?" "What kind of peanut butter?" "What kind of sliced ham?" "What kind of milk?" "Which kind of tuna?" Making these choices is part of the fun of the program. You and your kids are going to explore what works for you. When you buy ham, you are going to read labels and do a taste test. You may discover that you all love honey-baked ham for a reason. You may learn that yes, Jif peanut butter is yummy—because of the sugar content. The discovery of these details is just as much a part of the program as actually eating the foods. I want you to grope through this a bit. I want you and your children to be in a process of discovery with what you eat. And asking and answering these questions will contribute to your healing.

When you start off, you may not know what 1 ounce of cooked hamburger looks like. You may want to invest in a little kitchen scale and encourage your children to use it, or you can get an inexpensive postal scale at an office supply store. Either way, chose a digital model so even the younger ones can read it easily.

TO WEIGH OR NOT TO WEIGH

You have heard me say not to fret over numbers. Why a kitchen scale? It will help you and your children get a sense of basic protein portions. They can learn what 3 ounces of cooked hamburger looks like. Kids love to weigh their food, so the scale can add to kitchen fun. But remember, if the scale starts to make them crazy and they get caught in weighing and counting rather than listening and adapting, then get rid of it.

The grams-of-protein chart will give you a sense of why I always encourage the use of *dense* proteins like meat and chicken and fish. You get way more bang for the buck, so to speak. A child's stomach has a more limited capacity than an adult's. Using dense proteins gives you a way to amp up the level of protein in a small serving, without making a youngster feel overly full. As you look at this chart, you can also see the advantage of combining different protein sources to up the level. You will also notice that I have included some foods that you may not have thought of as breakfast foods. This is a way you and your children can have fun. Let them explore what suits them.

As you play with these ideas, you may wonder "Which sausage?" "What kind of chili?" "Should the cottage cheese be low fat? Large curd? Small curd?" "Which hot dogs?" "What kind of protein bar?" You may also notice that I am not being exact with brands or specific sizes. You are going to want me to give you specifics. But there is a very specific reason I am not. I want you and your children to find the answers to these questions yourselves. I want you to be reading labels and experimenting. You and the kids can make chili at home, or you can look at different brands of canned chili. The act of answering these questions is part of your healing. If I tell you, then it is "my" program you are doing. If you and your children go through this discovery, it becomes "your" program.

There is one more thing to remember. You may look at this list and wonder if I am out of my mind to suggest that a fast-food sausage-and-egg sandwich is a good alternative. After all, aren't those things high in fat and high in sodium? Yep, that's true—and they are a far sight better than pancakes and syrup. As you will see throughout this book, I am a very pragmatic woman. I am in touch with your real lives. People go to McDonald's. If I say to you, "Okay, regular meals, no white things, no sugar, no fast foods, no preservatives, no saturated fat, eat organic and home grown," you are going to smile politely and not be able to do that. When I talk about baby steps, I mean it. If I suggest putting whey protein powder into pancakes and using whole grain flour in your recipe, then you can make that change when you are ready so that it will work for your children. As they continue with the baby steps, they will feel empowered to make more. You will push your growing edge way more than I might suggest. And your kids will try even more. Let's take a look at some of my crazy combination breakfast options!

Sausage/Egg Sandwich		Burrito	
1 egg	6 g	¼ c. beans	4 g
1 slice cheese	5.5 g	1 slice cheese	5 g
1 sausage patty	8 g	1 oz. cooked hamburger	8 g
Total protein	19.5 g	Total protein	17 g
Chili		**Scrambled Eggs**	
½ c. beans	8 g	1 egg	6 g
2 oz. hamburger	12 g	cottage cheese	8 g
Total protein	20 g	4 oz. milk on the side	4 g
		Total protein	18 g
Yogurt Treat		**Cheese 'n' Dog**	
8 oz. yogurt	16 g	Cheese stick	6 g
1½ oz. sunflower seeds	10 g	Hot dog	8 g
Total protein	26 g	Total protein	14 g
Shake		**Peanut Butter Sandwich**	
½ scoop whey powder	8 g	3 tbsp. peanut butter	12 g
8 oz. milk	8 g	8 oz. milk	8 g
Total protein	16 g	Total protein	20 g
Protein Powder Pancakes		**Protein Bar Breakfast**	
⅓ batter w/3 scoops	16 g	Protein bar	12 g
2 oz. yogurt fruit spread	2 g	8 oz. milk	8 g
Total protein	26 g	Total protein	20 g

Have your children take a look at this list. Ask them to make up their own combinations. Don't be surprised if they come up with some combos you would have never imagined. This is the fun part. Kids teach us to think differently because they have not had years of conditioning over what a "proper" breakfast should be. Put the combinations and protein amounts you all come up with on some three-by-five index cards. Post them inside the kitchen cabinet to help you all remember what combinations will work for breakfast. Remember to choose foods that are appropriate for the age of your children. For instance, do not give nuts to children under three because they can choke on the pieces, and because you may increase the risk of an allergic reaction.

You may wonder which are the "best" proteins. The best proteins are the ones your child will eat. Perhaps you have heard that hot dogs are a "junk" food because they are high in fat and have a lot of additives. Or what about bologna, which is really just sliced huge hot dog? But if hot dogs and bologna are the only foods your three-year-old will touch, what are you to do? You do the best you can. Leave these questions and concerns until you are really settled on step seven of the program. Refinement and tweaking can come when you and your children are skilled with your food plan. For now, stick with hot dogs.

Using Protein Powders

Many parents have found that protein powder can be a lifesaver. You can use it to make protein shakes, or you can add it to things like pancakes and waffles. This is a wonderful way to increase the protein intake for your children. For example, if a recipe calls for 2 cups of all-purpose flour, try using 1 cup each of whey protein powder and flour. Try adding extra powder to pancakes, waffles, biscuits, egg bakes, quiche, and cookies. If you are making baked goods, you can replace up to half the flour content with a protein powder. Begin experimenting by adding 1 scoop (about ¼ cup) at a time. Whisk it thoroughly to avoid lumps. You might want to use a hand blender or a food processor to mix liquids or batters, particularly if you are making a creamy soup, dressing, or sauce. If your recipe starts getting too thick, don't panic; simply add more liquid to adjust the consistency.

Different protein powders have different textures and will affect your recipes in different ways. Do not use soy-based powders or soymilk with children. I know that soy products and soymilk are being widely marketed to children, but in fact, the estrogenic properties of soy can have a hormonal effect on growing bodies. Increased estrogen levels can cause girls to have an early puberty and boys to grow breasts. Occasional use of soy is fine, but not daily and not in large amounts. Whey protein powder is a far better alternative for children. Whey protein is a product made from milk. The proteins are distilled by passing the milk through a series of filters with different-size holes. The end result is very pure and concentrated. Even many children who have a problem with dairy can tolerate whey protein powder because it is so distilled. Whey protein powder is also rich in something called alpha-lactalbumin, which increases the level of tryptophan in the brain. Increasing the tryptophan level enhances the serotonin levels as well. More serotonin means less depression and more impulse control. Most children really like whey protein powders, but it is important for you to experiment with different brands. Check the label to make sure you are getting a sweetener-free product. Do not use a product with aspartame.

The serotonin-enhancing quality of lactalbumin-rich

whey encouraged me to choose it for use in our own children's shake product called George's Jr.—an adaptation of our famous George's Shake. It is made with a form of protein that is very bioavailable, which means the protein is easy to digest and quickly absorbed. You can get the shake mix from our website at www.radiantrecovery.com or purchase your own whey protein powder at a natural foods store. George's Jr. has no sweeteners added, no sugar, and no other added ingredients or added sweeteners like aspartame, Splenda, potassium aspartate, maltitol, or brown rice syrup. It has a mild neutral flavor so your children can add fruit, like half a frozen banana or some nonalcohol-based natural flavorings like coconut and orange. We have added a number of different nonalcohol-based flavorings to our website store, so each of your children can have a shake to his or her personal taste.

A whey shake in the morning works really well, especially for kids who are not big on breakfast. It is quick and tasty, and it has a big protein bang for the buck. If you are making a shake, the best option is George's Jr. My four-year-old granddaughter is a very picky eater. Pancakes and syrup are her preferred breakfast choice. When she comes for a visit, we need to find other alternatives. She loves to help cook. I put the blender on the table so she can easily reach it from the chair. I open a carton of oat milk (a grain-based "milk" that I use in my own shake), take the lid off the apple juice container, and get out the whey protein powder and some oatmeal. I get out a ¼ cup measure, the measuring spoons, and a set of tiny measuring spoons labeled a "pinch," a "smidgen," and a "dash."

"Okay, Madison, I want you to put a quarter cup of oat milk in the blender." I help her pour the oat milk into the blender. Then we add the apple juice. She measures a tablespoon of George's Jr. protein powder mix. Then I asked her what flavor shake she wants. She decides on orange coconut, so she pours a "pinch" from the bottles of flavoring and puts them in her shake. She puts the lid on the blender, turns it on, lets it whir, and chooses a cup. I help her pour it into her cup. She drinks it all. Most significant, the next day she comes in and says, "Namo, may I make some more of that apple milk?" So we do. The idea of breakfast with protein is forming in her brain.

GEORGE'S JR. SHAKE

*1 cup **liquid** (Use milk, oat milk, almond milk, or rice milk when you are starting. Later you can use part milk and part juice. Apple juice seems to work best.)*

***George's Jr. Mix** (It has both protein and complex carbohydrate in it.) Amount depends on your child's size. Check the label.*

*Frozen **fruit** to taste (Use half a frozen banana, frozen strawberries, or frozen peaches. If you get frozen fruit at the store, use the fruit with no sweetener added.)*

Flavoring as preferred if you don't use fruit.

Blend for 30 seconds on high.

Let your children be outrageous. They may want chili on a hamburger bun for breakfast. They may want leftover pizza. Tell them what is totally negotiable, what is not. Chili works, no breakfast doesn't. (And remember, mom has to do this as well. You don't get to help them with breakfast and then go off for your latte without eating. At each step you will be doing it right along with them. One of our community members, Vicki, has "pancake grandchildren" like I do. She simply adds whey powder to the pancake mix and makes pancakes with sausage, applesauce, and yogurt. They love it. Refer to the chapter on recipes, beginning on page 211. I have included a number of very child-friendly choices—including some things your kids can make themselves. Sausage and Egg Bake (page 225) or Dutch Puffed Pancakes (page 222) are yummy and easy to prepare.

As I said earlier, children have small stomachs, so you should strive for what I call "dense" proteins—literally, those that you can hold in your hand, as opposed to items like milk and yogurt. Try using cheese and meats when you can. Cottage cheese is ideal. Some children love it, and some children won't touch it. Try different brands, as they have very different textures and smells. As you look at the protein list on page 60, you can see that eggs and meat are very efficient protein carriers.

> *I have started cutting out pictures of foods from magazines so that we can put together a handy reference guide of foods with protein. My goal is to have a page of protein-based breakfast options that [my child] can choose each morning (scrambled eggs and wheat toast, oatmeal with protein powder, cottage cheese and fruit).*
>
> *Jennifer*

If you take the time to teach your children how to count grams of protein, even the little ones will get it. Sometimes moving out of the traditional breakfast box will do wonders for the picky eaters in your family. Some families create a "breakfast bar." The kids come up with the options, mom gives them a budget and the funds, and they shop for the items. Some families set up a shake bar, some a cereal bar with hard-boiled eggs. They all end up being able to have what works for each person. It is an ideal solution. You might try making the Apple Ham Bake Breakfast (page 224) and setting it out for them to have as much as they like.

> *I started having my kids fix their own breakfasts when they were pretty young. My six-year-old son would fry himself eggs in the morning (of course he had to stand on the chair to do it). Now he is fixing himself ham and cheese omelets!*
>
> *Dianne*

If you have a picky eater in your house, don't be discouraged. Go slowly, let them pick. Have them talk with you about what it is that bothers them. Taste? Texture? Smell? And trust that as you do the food plan, "picky" often disappears. I have found a huge correlation between sugar consumption and "picky." Little sugar addicts like white things and sweet things, not green things and brown things. Be patient. This will change.

If you are reading this and planning, you may be thinking, "Yeah, Kathleen, this is a great idea, but you don't know what it's like in our house. No one will get out of bed on time, kids dawdle. The only thing that works is TV. It keeps them timed. Gotta be dressed by one *Sponge Bob,* and we leave after the second one."

Be creative. Give them a shake with *Sponge Bob.* Have them put shake-enriched milk on their cereal while watching *Sponge Bob* or whatever they regularly watch.

Hand them a shake in the car. Give them a whole grain bagel with peanut butter to munch on the bus. Wrap up the scrambled eggs in a whole wheat tortilla. Don't be a purist. Strive for baby steps that work.

Adding Carbohydrates

Once you have mastered the protein phase of breakfast, start thinking about the carbohydrate phase—protein and carbohydrate at every breakfast. Over time you are going to shift from "white" carbohydrates to "brown" carbohydrates. In making that shift with children, I often suggest moving toward "beige" first. We will talk in more depth about "browning" your family in step five, but for now just be attentive. Make sure breakfast includes something like protein *and* waffles, pancakes, cereals like Cheerios, Shredded Wheat, Grape-Nuts, homemade granola, or oatmeal, rice cakes, bagels, English muffins, or whole grain toast. If you can, move toward cereals with less than 10 grams of sugar per serving. Have your kids read labels. Have them go on a cereal quest at the store. Make sure to go shopping when they are not tired and hungry. Have the seven-year-old take the three-year-old to look for stuff. Let them have fun, and they will love it.

Putting It Together

As *you* do breakfast, everyone is going to feel better. Just that one change will have a huge impact on you and your children. If *you* are having breakfast, you will be more focused and time will expand. The key is not to try to do any more than breakfast right now. Not taking out the sugar, not being a Norman Rockwell family, not striving for perfection. The only thing that matters is having breakfast, on time, enough, and in the right balance. Ask your children to problem-solve with you. You will be astounded at how creative they are.

> *I am working on letting my children have some control in their own food choices, instead of me making the choices. This has been hard. . . . The only thing they know about sugar sensitivity is what I tell them. By not experiencing it themselves, they don't really know what I'm talking about. I think this will further add to their "protection."*
>
> Gail

The children themselves may take their program beyond what you imagine for them. Here is a recipe for pancakes that eight-year-old Sacha sent from Portsmouth, England. Her invention has about 15 grams of protein in one serving. For each person use:

1 tablespoon whole wheat flour
1 tablespoon cottage cheese
1 egg
2 tablespoons milk

Whiz all the ingredients in blender until smooth. Poor/spoon the mixture onto a hot frying pan, and cook like a normal pancake. Don't worry about the cottage cheese. I didn't think it would be nice, but you don't notice it is there!

We asked our online community parents to share what their children were eating. Remember, these are the kids who used to eat sugar cereals and Pop-Tarts.

- oatmeal and eggs on the side
- quiche with eggs, cheese, and veggies, made the night before
- homemade sugar-free baked beans and hot dogs
- cheese and whole wheat bread
- pancakes with extra eggs and protein powder
- whole wheat tortillas with scrambled eggs, ham, and cheese
- cottage cheese with fruit and whole grain English muffins
- cheese quesadillas with ham or turkey
- burritos made with corn tortillas, beans, cheese, and chicken
- whole grain cereal with cheese sticks on the side
- six-egg omelet, split with all the kids
- poached eggs in cups
- leftover pizza with sausage on the side
- apples and peanut butter
- leftovers from last night's dinner
- pancakes made from eggs and raw oatmeal
- "toads in a hole" (cooked eggs in the middle of whole grain toast)

One parent sent in a custard recipe that many of our kids and parents just love. The total recipe has about 65 grams of protein. Three one-cup servings would give you a little more than 20 grams per serving. Six half-cup servings would give you a little more than 10 grams per serving. Here it is:

3 cups milk (cow, oat, almond, or other non-soy alternatives)
¾ cup nonfat powdered milk
3 eggs
½ teaspoon vanilla
dash of nutmeg

1. Preheat the oven to 350°F. Combine the milk and powdered milk in a saucepan over medium heat. Bring to a low boil, stirring constantly.

2. Beat the eggs in a small bowl, add the vanilla, and stir into the heated milk slowly.

3. Pour into half-cup-size custard cups that have been lightly buttered, sprinkle with nutmeg, place in a shallow pan of water, and bake for 40 minutes.

Serves 6

As you look at the community parents' list on page 72, you can see that your children can prepare almost any of these breakfasts. Many parents and children make up a batch of what they want for the week and keep it in the refrigerator or freezer. Homemade protein waffles replace Pop-Tarts in the toaster at seven A.M. Easy Egg and Oat One-Pan Breakfast (page 224) is simple enough for a six-year-old to make. Share the list with your children. Ask them which things sound good to them. Let them go shopping for the stuff. Let them experiment on the weekend so they can try things out when they are not rushed. Let them copy the list of breakfast options to take to Dad's house so they can make a program-friendly breakfast there as well. Have them e-mail the recipe for protein pancakes to your mother so she can get what they need for their next visits. Fun is the key word here.

My daughter (first grade) was having problems in school. The teacher said she thought Sarah was ADD or ADHD. She said Sarah would twirl her hair and get in a hypnotic state and not be able to focus in class. I made changes in her diet like no more sugary cereal for breakfast, no pancakes without protein, and things like that. I notice a huge difference in her behavior at home, and amazingly enough she doesn't twirl her hair anymore.

Lee

Bumps Along the Way

Despite your best efforts, some children may balk at eating within an hour of getting up. They may say they are not hungry, or that it makes them feel sick, or that they just can't bear it. Generally these are girls, often small and slender girls. It is true that some children are simply not morning children and the idea of food first thing just sets them off. But it is also true that not eating creates a specific biochemical response. When the body goes into not-eating mode, it releases beta-endorphin to protect the brain from knowing it is starving. The beta-endorphin makes your child feel good, mean and lean and able to cope. The child likes this feeling and learns that not-eating evokes it. This not-eating in order to feel good (or pretty) is one of the earliest clues that your child may be at risk for an eating disorder. Pay very close attention to this dynamic. If left alone, it can quickly take her down a serious path of anorexic eating patterns. Your job is to intervene early on in such a way that the biochemical pattern is not set up.

In the beginning, simply work with your child to find a solution that is tolerable. Sometimes a chocolate shake with whey protein powder is a good start. Once your child starts to eat something, this pattern will change. The "I can't eat" feeling comes from a nausea that is a result of low blood sugar. So even though it feels like food is the last thing in the world they want, food is the very thing that they need most and that will heal the problem. Give these children some protein before they go to bed. A protein snack will maintain blood sugar levels longer, and they will not wake up in such crisis in the morning.

Another problem may be that Daddy or your partner does not eat breakfast, so your kids get contradictory messages about the importance of breakfast. If the children ask you about it, you might say with a smile, "And look how cranky Daddy is!" Or, "Daddy gets to make his own mistakes. He is grown up. I am not in charge of his health. But I am in charge of yours." You say it with a smile. Don't make Daddy look bad, just tell the kids it is not negotiable for you and them. You can say it is Daddy's choice but they don't have a choice. It is not your job to fix the other adult members of the household. It is your job to guide your children into good health. Just tell them that. They may grumble, but they will get it.

If you are divorced or separated, they may go to Daddy's house, where you have no control over breakfast or food. You do the best you can. You may have the same dilemma at your mother's or mother-in-law's house. Just ask them to have what you need on hand. Send them some recipes or this book. Highlight this chapter. Ask them to help. If you have a sense of humor and detachment about it, it will work better. And stash a Baggie of protein powder in the suitcase when you go. (Don't try this if you travel by plane. It may be confiscated!)

I hope you now understand the gist of my approach toward breakfast. Humor, participation, unfailing insistence, and consistency will work. And after a month of breakfast, you will be thrilled at what change this one step has created.

4

Step Two:
Making Connections

When you did your detective work back in Chapter 2, you had the experience of making connections between what and when your children were eating and how they felt. Now I want you to help guide your children through a process of making their *own* connections. Most children never know that what and when they eat makes a *huge* difference in how they feel. They don't know that sugary cereal for breakfast makes them cranky at school. They don't know that sugary cereal at breakfast makes them funny for an hour and then really sleepy.

The first job you will do is to help them notice what they eat. This is Step Two—Making Connections. Take them to get a little notebook just for this. We call it a food journal, but you can call it a diary or a record book, or you can let your children name the book. Let the children choose books that suit them. Each child in your family will need a different book. Ask each child to use it for four days to write down what he or she eats and at what time.

If they are really little and have not learned to write, you will need to help them. They can draw pictures or use stickers to record their meals and snacks. We will start by looking at breakfast. This is the part of the program you and your children are most skilled at. Over time you and they will generalize toward all the meals.

Show the kids specifically how to make the entries. Have them make a notation of each meal. Then teach them to look at the clock, see what time it is, and write down the time and then what they had. Help them be as detailed as they can, and if they are old enough to note actual amounts of food ("a cup of milk" rather than just "some milk"), that's even better. But don't fret about the numbers. The process is what counts most. Writing about breakfast might look like this:

6:30 A.M.   A Pop-Tart and a glass of chocolate milk
             or
7 A.M.   A bowl of frosted shredded wheat and a
             little glass of orange juice
             or maybe
8 A.M.   An Egg McMuffin, potatoes, and a Coke

Encourage them to be honest, and help them remember. Don't judge their comments or choices. Even if they had ice cream and leftover birthday cake, that is okay. Just have them write it down. Suggest they write down their foods as soon as they eat them (or close to the time), not at the end of the day, as they may not remember. Support the process of recording. Help them understand the nuances of journaling like adding comments about time or other things that were going on. The journal could say:

7 A.M.   We were late for school and forgot breakfast
          or
7 A.M.   Just had time for a banana and granola bar in
          the car

Talk to them about writing down feelings as well. Give
them a little index card with feeling words to put in their
journals. Ask them to write down the feelings they think
fit them. Brainstorm with all your children and see what
you come up with. The card might say

HAPPY	FUNNY	RELAXED
MAD	WHINY	JUMPY
GRUMPY	SCARED	TIRED

Tell them you are just starting by gathering four days of
information, and then you will all play with the data they
gather. Tony is ten. Here is a picture of Tony's record
book. Show this to them so they can see what Tony wrote.

Monday 7 A.M.	Big bowl of Cheerios and milk	Tired. Hard to get up Mad at Mom
9:30 A.M. 10:00 A.M.	Granola bar at recess	Really hungry Feel better
11:30 A.M.	Pizza and soda	Feel really good Funny and goofy with my friends
1:00 P.M.		Really tired
2:30 P.M.	Candy bar on way home	So hungry I wanted to eat everything Mad at everybody
3:15 P.M.	2 peanut butter and jelly sandwiches	Want to take a nap

| 6:00 P.M. | Hamburger
Corn
Fries
Glass of milk | Having a good time |
| 8:00 P.M. | | Tired and cranky |

Tony loves to play sports so he thought of his book as a training record. He did a great job. Give your children the message that they can use whatever style works for them. Give them a lot of energy over the next four days—lots of positive support and enthusiasm. See how they are doing. Show them your own food journal. Do yours on the dining room table with them there so they can get the idea of how to do it. If you do it together, it will be more fun.

Each day ask questions like "How did you do? Did you remember to write things down? Was it really hard, or was it fun?" Talk, talk, talk about it. Don't nag, and keep it fun. Share what you are experiencing with your kids.

If the kids will do this for four days, they will learn a lot. Now your job is to help them see the meaning in what they have been recording. Creating meaning is what makes the journal process come alive. If you present this step as an investigation into what makes them tick, they will start making connections between what and when they eat and how they feel.

Here are some more questions to ask your kids that are designed to help make the connections. Don't interrogate them, and don't judge. This is really important: sugar sensitive children are very intuitive and will know what you are feeling. If your mouth says, "That's great, Tim," and your body says, "Oh, help! I can't believe you eat this way!" he will know. Do not send conflicting messages. If it is hard for you not to judge, share that. Be funny. And share your own journal. It will help keep you "clean." Don't ask all these questions, of course. Pick a couple that seem to fit your child, and find a peaceful time in the day to have this discussion. Ask the questions over the course of a few days. Note that these questions all focus on breakfast as the starting point because that is the meal your children will now have the most experience with.

Do you have breakfast every morning?

Some kids are really surprised that they forget to eat breakfast some days. They are late for school, run out the door, and just forget. Does this happen to you at all? Who makes your breakfasts? Is your breakfast different on the weekends?

What time do you have it?

Do you have it early or later? Is it hard for you to wake up, or do you jump out of bed? Are you hungry in the morning, or do you hate the idea of eating?

Do you have breakfast within an hour of getting out of bed?

This one is important to notice. Do you get busy and forget? Do you run off to play and not notice the time? What happens with the time between getting up and having breakfast?

What do you usually have for breakfast?

Is it the same each morning? Do you get tired of the same, or do you like it? Is it too much, or do you wish you could eat more and more?

Do you like breakfast?

Do you hop out of bed thinking, "Oh, boy, *breakfast!*" or do you go, "Ugh, breakfast again!" and feel bad?

What is your favorite breakfast?

Write down your most favorite breakfast in the world. What would you eat, and whom would you eat it with?

Do you have different things for breakfast on school days and on weekends?

Why? Why not? Who decides this?

Do you sit down for breakfast, or do you eat it standing up or riding in the car?

It's fun to realize where and how you eat. Some kids eat in front of the TV while they're watching *Sponge Bob.* Their mom tells them, "You have to finish by the first *Sponge Bob,* and you have to be ready to go by the second *Sponge Bob.*" Think about what we do in our house.

Do you have breakfast by yourself, or do you eat with your family?

I bet you never thought of this before. A lot of times kids just have cereal alone while everyone else is getting ready.

How is it in our family? Do you like how it is, or would you like a change?

Who chooses what you get for breakfast?

Do you choose, or does a grown-up choose for you? Do you get to say what you like? Do you have a fit if you don't get what you want? Do you ever refuse to eat it if you don't like it? What happens if you get mad about your breakfast?

Do you get enough to eat, or would you like more?

Sometimes kids would like four bowls of cereal, but Mom or Dad only lets them have one. Does this ever happen to you? Do you want to eat more and don't? Is mealtime a happy time for you?

How much sugar do you eat at breakfast?

You can figure this out by looking on the box of your cereal or on the bread wrapper. Cereals are very different in how much sugar they have in one serving. When you are figuring this out, you have to really pay attention to what a serving size is. One serving might have 15 grams of sugar, but the size of the serving is half a cup. If you have a big bowl, you might be having three times that amount, so you are really getting 45 grams of sugar.

Here is the fun part. You are going to do a little experiment to see what the stated grams of sugar would look like in actual piles of sugar. Have your children read labels and count how many grams of sugar they get in a typical breakfast. Four grams equals 1 teaspoon of sugar. If you had 40 grams of sugar for breakfast, that would be the same as having 10 teaspoons of sugar.

Get out the measuring spoons, the sugar bowl, and a piece of paper towel. Have the kids measure out the number of teaspoons of sugar they had for breakfast on the paper towel. Let them make a pile so they can see how big it is. Does the size of the pile surprise them?

Now here is some more fun math to do. The effect of the sugar changes depending on how much they weigh. Let's think of the sugar as a dose of a drug. Here is an experiment to see what this means.

Measure out 10 teaspoons of sugar. This is the same amount of sugar in a can of soda. Get a little glass that holds about one cup. Get a big container that holds a quart or a liter. Put 10 teaspoons in each container and then fill it with water. Now taste the difference. Which is sweeter?

The little one will be way sweeter because it is more sugar and less water. Let your children get that their bodies are the same as the containers. If little sister weighs only 30 pounds and has a soda, it will affect her much more than it will affect the one who is 90 pounds. In fact, it will be three times more powerful. This kind of experimentation can get the concept over way more powerfully than your telling them that sugar is bad will ever do. Because your children now have some experience with counting food grams, the concept is going to make sense to them. Now they have a magic number. Your job is to support them in figuring how they will get what they need.

As gathering data progresses, you will also be making other kinds of connections. You and your children are going to start noticing the relationship between eating and behavior. Let me share a personal story that powerfully brought this home to me.

My daughter and her two boys, aged seven and three, were driving with me from Southboro, Massachusetts, to Long Island, New York. It was nearly a three-hour drive, and it was late in the day. The little one was in his car seat and starting to fall apart. It was raining and dark, and there was glare on the road. We were driving past construction barriers on the side of the road and could not pull over. The three-year-old had eaten a lot of sweet stuff at the family reunion we had attended earlier in the day. He started screaming, "I want you to pick me up," kicking, howling, and saying the same thing over and over. He was totally out of control. When he gets in that place, it is like being caught in a groove he cannot rationally get out of. Reasoning does not help. Blankie doesn't help. He screamed for an hour and a half.

I watched my daughter get grayer and grayer. She was concentrating on driving and simply went into an altered state to cope with the rain and the construction barriers. I watched my feelings and noticed what kind of energy it took to disassociate. What a struggle! If we stopped and picked him up, were we reinforcing his behavior? If we didn't, were we allowing the "abuse" he was putting on us? But he was locked in a loop and nothing would shift the cycle.

Finally, the seven-year-old, who had been playing with his GameBoy for all that time (also in an altered state), screamed at him and smacked him, "Tyler, *stop* it!" Then, of course, Mom screamed at the seven-year-old. I was trying to stay out of it. But interestingly, the smack pushed his brother out of the groove, and now he was simply cry-ing rather than screaming obsessively. So Mom suggested the older one give his brother some water. He did. We had simple sniffling the rest of the way.

When we got to New York, it was late and my daughter was about to fall apart. I could feel it. I told her that I would put the little one to bed so she could have a break. I cleaned him up, got his PJs on, and soothed him. He was asleep in about ten minutes.

His behavior was about chemistry, not about personal-ity. Food creates a whole cascade of behaviors and dynam-ics—which we assume are about personality. We forget that food started the behavior, and before we know it, we end up with therapy and patterns and assumptions about who kids are. But the behavior is connected to the food.

This experience in the car made me reflect on what I could have done. That morning, while Mom slept, I had taken the boys out for a good breakfast of eggs and pota-toes, no cinnamon rolls or syrupy pancakes. But I did not think to go into the little country store and get some "stash" for the drive—almonds, cheese sticks, fruit. I didn't say to my daughter, "Hey Jen, I bet there's going to be *lots* of sweet stuff at the reunion. Shall we plan how to handle it? How can I support you? I have some snacks." I needed to remember that it is impossible to make connec-tions about food and mood when you are in the middle of a meltdown. I forgot the first rule of making connections. Assume the problem is the food first, and think of it as a biochemical problem to be solved, not an out-of-control child. Had I remembered this rule, I would have said, "Let's pull over and find a snack and help him calm down."

Because we have a little distance, grandparents can be really helpful in learning to do the food. We can provide a different kind of support. We can carry a stash of good stuff like cheese instead of the cookies that subvert their process. We can learn new ways right along with the kids.

5

Step Three:
Snacks and Drinks

Having a regular breakfast with protein is the first step in healing the volatile blood sugar of sugar sensitivity. Making connections is the second, and having regular, substantive snacks is the third step. Maintaining a stable blood sugar is significantly more important in children than in adults, and I think it is easy for parents to miss this. Many sugar sensitive children and parents graze through the day. This eating can be unconscious and most often drifts to carbohydrates. In this chapter, you are going to make an intentional commitment to planning snacks and to paying attention to what your child is drinking, especially soda.

Snacks

Now that you and your children have a good sense of what protein foods are, it will be relatively easy to identify good protein foods for snacks. Make each snack a combination of protein and carbohydrates. Plan for snacks. Ideally, growing children need something at midmorning and mid-afternoon. Your child should not go more than three hours without having something to eat. Here are some of the snacks our community parents give their children:

- an apple or Triscuits (whole wheat crackers) and some cheese
- a few whole grain crackers with a mozzarella stick or sliced cheese
- a hard-boiled egg with a handful of carrot sticks
- a slice of whole wheat toast with "old-fashioned" peanut butter (the variety with no added sugar, made with just peanuts)
- a handful of nuts (for children over age three)
- cottage cheese and some unsweetened canned pineapple
- applesauce and leftover sausage
- leftover Apple Ham Bake Breakfast (see page 224)
- a cup of chili heated in the microwave and two corn tortillas
- a bean or meat burrito
- a snack mix made with pumpkin seeds, peanuts, Wheat Chex, and Cheerios mixed together and baked with some light olive oil
- tacos with warmed hamburger, cheese, chopped tomato, and lettuce
- a peanut butter and fruit spread sandwich on whole grain bread

If your child's school does not presently allow snacks at midmorning, ask them if they will. Talk to the teacher.

You may find she is more supportive than you expect. Give her a copy of this book or a copy of the snack list. Tell her what you are trying to do. Be specific and suggest snack alternatives other than the usual cookies or cupcakes. Have your children help you make a list of possibilities to share with her. Ask her if she might do a unit on healthy snacks with the children in the class. You might find that she is right on the same page with you and will love having you as an ally. I cannot tell you how often things that are classified by teachers as behavior problems simply go away when children maintain an adequate blood sugar level. Whining, pouting, fighting, not paying attention, talking back, being spacey, throwing temper tantrums, and being defiant and stubborn can all be a function of low blood sugar.

Here is what Elaine, a member of our community who also happens to be a teacher, said:

> I asked my kids what they had for breakfast today. I was appalled to hear what they had to say. Candy, cookies, cake. Unbelievable. I decided right then and there to send home a paper today asking the parents to write what the children have for breakfast tomorrow. It's part of their homework. I feel like making hard-boiled eggs or getting string cheese to hand them as they walk in the door. I can't afford to do that every day, but I sure would like to. I would love to see the difference in how they behave and learn. I wonder if I could get a grant to study this!!! OY!

See what you can do to get teachers and other parents on your side. You might raise the issue of snacks at a PTA meeting. Be bold, and do not assume you are the only one concerned about this issue. But don't wait for the school to change—start with your own child. Ask her how snacks can be worked into the school day. Ask her what she can take in her backpack that won't be messy to eat. String cheese and individually packaged crackers are great.

Many of our parents have tried different approaches to discipline when their children exhibit whining, fighting, and the other "bad" behaviors. These approaches include all the typical interventions you have heard of: time-outs, warnings, taking away privileges—all the things the experts tell us to do. They also sometimes include things that the experts tell us not to do, like yelling and smacking. Unless you address the food issues, however, neither discipline nor punishment will work with sugar sensitive children. Little sugar addicts are in an altered state when their chemistry is off. They are not rational. If you can begin to look at these "bad" behaviors in a new way, you may be able to come up with some creative alternatives for what to do if your little sugar sensitive child starts acting up. First of all, feed him. Give him some protein and fruit right away. The fruit will deal with any sugar withdrawal that might be operating and will provide quick blood sugar relief. The protein will provide sustained, time-release support to his blood sugar.

We have a funny saying in our parent community— "Cheese, not soap." A cheese stick does wonders for a mouthy kid. Keep cheese sticks in the refrigerator all the time. Carry almonds in your purse. Put some of the dehydrated cheese snacks we carry in our store (at www. radiantrecovery.com) in the glove compartment. Know what choices are available in the local gas station mart.

Things like cheese, crackers, and hard-boiled eggs can save a child whose blood sugar is falling. Always have some power food available. If you are running errands, know where to stop for the right snacks, and feed your child in an emergency.

> Yesterday my thirteen-year-old did not do his chores right, and when I asked him to finish them correctly, he said, "Mom, what do you expect? It is not my fault that I forgot to finish—it's my messed-up biochemistry." My kids are too smart for me—but I was able to counter him by tossing him a cheese stick. And it worked. Today I noticed my husband giving the kids protein. And even better, telling the kids to wait for a sugar treat until after dinner. Sometimes I think I need to stop thinking so much and just start doing. My husband did not need the whole theory, he just thought it made sense and gave it a try. I think I can learn from this.
>
> DeAnna

Feed your children when they come home from school. They cannot go from noon till six without food. Their metabolism simply cannot cope for that amount of time. If you are home, fix them something. If you work and they are responsible for after-school fare, make sure to stock up and leave sufficient choices for them. Many children do really well with leftovers. We call the leftovers you intentionally make for the next day "planned overs." If you make extra and have planned overs, you can make it really easy for your children to snack when they get home.

For children who play after-school sports, a planned snack is even more important. Pack an extra sandwich.

Send along shake mix in a plastic bag. Your child can get an extra carton of milk and mix it with the protein powder. Or you can get some dry milk powder and mix it with the protein powder, put it in a shaker cup, and stash it in the backpack.

Many parents send sandwiches with lunch meat or peanut butter for after-school snacks. Go back and look again at the chart showing the protein amounts children need on page 60. Generally speaking, shoot for a snack to contain half the protein that a meal would contain. If your child needs 20 grams of protein for breakfast, she will need 10 grams for her snack. A slice of bologna has about 3 grams, so it may not be the best choice. Most parents, as they do these calculations, realize that the snacks they have been providing are low in protein.

As you plan snacks with your children, beware of seemingly "healthy" options like sweetened dried fruit or fruit "roll-ups." These items are mainly concentrated sugar. The chewier the fruit, the more concentrated the sugar. If you give your children eight pieces of dried apricot, you are giving them the equivalent of four whole pieces of fruit. This same thing is true of raisins. Whole fruits are best because of the vitamins, minerals, and fiber they contain. Have fruit with protein. An apple and some cheese. Cottage cheese and pineapple.

If you choose snack bars or protein bars, read the labels. Many are packed with sugars—one brand has twelve different forms of sugar. The manufacturers use different names for sugar so that *sugar* does not have to show as the first and primary ingredient. I once did a really fun experiment with a group of schoolchildren. We collected protein bar labels, took them to the copy store, and got them enlarged. Then we compared all the different kinds of sugars we found. Most bars have 30 grams of sugars. Find the ones with less, and have your children taste them. Here is the catch. Usually the ones with lower sugar taste like pressed cardboard. Making your own "power bars" can be really fun. Try making our Radiant Snack Bars (recipe below). Make your own trail mix with nuts, minus the dried fruit, and send it with fresh fruit. Or try this idea: Mix raw rolled oats (I use Quaker's Instant in the big cylinder) with peanut butter and whole fruit jelly, and spread the mixture onto waxed paper; roll it into a sausage shape and refrigerate. When the "dough" hardens enough, you can slice off "cookies" in desired amounts. You can play with the ratio of oats to peanut butter and jelly depending on your kids' tastes.

RADIANT SNACK BARS

6 cups	rolled oats (one cylindrical container)
1 dozen	eggs
½ cup	cinnamon
4 cups	liquid (milk, oat milk, or juice of your choice)
1 cup	cottage cheese or whey protein powder
2 cups	shredded unsweetened coconut, lightly toasted
1 teaspoon	salt
	Additional ½ cup shredded unsweetened coconut for topping

Blend the wet ingredients for 1 minute.

Mix the dry ingredients together in a large bowl.

Add the liquid mixture to the dry ingredients a little at a time until thoroughly mixed.

RADIANT SNACK BARS *(continued)*

Pour into a 9-by-13-inch pan that has been sprayed with cooking spray.

Sprinkle an additional ½ cup unsweetened coconut on top. (Don't toast it.)

Bake 1 hour at 350°F.

Let cool and slice into "bars" that are sized for your children.

You can add other things like nuts or sliced apples if you like. Experiment. Your family may like a different texture. Adjust the liquid, and try different options. This is a recipe to "play" with.

A number of people have reported seeing a huge change in their child's attitude just from this one change of adding regular protein/carbohydrate snacks. Getting enough to eat at regular intervals is crucial for the sugar sensitive child. Maintaining a stable blood sugar level is significantly more important in children than in adults, something I think it is easy for parents to miss.

Drinks

As you began your discovery of your children's typical eating patterns in Chapter 2, you may have learned that drinking soda is high on the list of favorites. Don't feel badly if your children are regular soda drinkers. One-fifth of all two-year-old children in our country are drinking almost a cup of soda a day. Children between six and eleven usually drink 15 ounces a day, and teens often drink almost 30 ounces a day. So your kids are in good company. Soda manufacturers do a powerful job of advertising. The four major soda companies spent $631 million on advertising in 1997. Coca-Cola is paying $60 million over ten years to the Boys & Girls Clubs of America to have exclusive market rights in the two thousand clubs. According to information provided to shareholders, Coca-Cola says it wants to:

> Make Coca-Cola the preferred drink for any occasion, whether it's a simple family supper or a formal state dinner . . . to build pervasiveness of our products, we are putting ice cold Coca-Cola Classic and our other brands within reach, wherever you look, at the supermarket, the video store, the soccer field, the gas station—everywhere.

So the amount of soda your children drink is not just a function of you. They are the targets of a major market thrust from the large soda makers. My concern with soda is twofold: it is liquid candy, and it is laced with caffeine. Let me talk with you about the seriousness of each of these. I will talk about caffeine first because you may be less aware of its impact.

Caffeine

Many parents do not know how powerful a drug caffeine is because caffeine is a part of their lives as well. And because caffeine operates like most drugs, you build a tolerance for it over time. As this happens, you do not notice its effects. As the former Queen of Caffeine, I used to hold the position that a little of it was fine. Having morning tea and an occasional "half caf" latte seemed to have no effect. However, I began to experience a persistent rapid heart rate. My own doctor was baffled and never considered caffeine as the cause. One morning I woke up with a caffeine withdrawal headache and had an insight. Maybe the caffeine was causing my rapid heartbeat. I stopped using caffeine, and the problem vanished. Here are some of the interesting facts I have learned abut caffeine.

- Caffeine is a *drug*. Its effect peaks in 40–60 minutes, and it takes 3–7 hours to get it out of your system. It passes into breast milk, amniotic fluid, fetal tissue, and semen. Newborns do not clear it well because they have not developed the enzymes that take it out of the body. If you are breastfeeding, your baby may not be sleeping because of the caffeine you are drinking.
- Caffeine works by blocking a neurotransmitter called adenosine that quiets your brain. By knocking it out, the net effect is the pleasant stimulation you feel when you use it. Caffeine also increases your levels of epinephrine, norepineprine, and serum cortisol. This drives the heart rate up and increases the "stress" response in the body. Increasing the stress response contributes to insulin resistance and weight gain when caffeine is used in a diet with lots of sugar (i.e., in soda).
- Caffeine contributes to sleep disturbance by blocking a brain chemical called GABA that is responsible for putting your brain to sleep. It is as if GABA has the job of singing you a lullaby, and caffeine comes busting into the room and flips on the radio to hard rock.
- Caffeine makes urinary incontinence worse. If you are a grown-up, this means getting up several times a

night to pee. If you are a child, it means wetting the bed.

- Caffeine also causes an increase in serotonin receptors that causes the serotonin factory to think there is less need to produce it. The net effect is a reduction in the production of the critical brain chemical that affects something called impulse control. Lots of caffeine makes it hard to "just say no."

All this science aside, I found some moving evidence about the impact of caffeine in the work of a researcher supported by the National Science Foundation, Peter Witt. Witt gave a group of spiders different drugs in the late '60s. He used spiders that make what is called an orb web—a web that is beautiful, highly regular and predictable, and easily photographed. I have always been very touched by the beauty of orb spiderwebs. I was recently in a train station in Harrisburg, Pennsylvania at night. There was a web just like the one pictured opposite, covered with raindrops, glistening in the light from the lamp on the platform. It was breathtaking.

Witt gave his orb web spiders LSD, marijuana, amphetamine, and caffeine to see if the drugs would affect how they made webs. Here is Witt's picture of a web made by a spider on caffeine. Sort of stops you cold, doesn't it? It's a very powerful visual of what might be happening in our own brains when we take drugs. I keep thinking about what it might mean for a child's ability to organize his thoughts. I keep wondering how much of what we diagnose as ADD is really caffeine-disorganized brains. So part of our healing story is to look at how much caffeine your child is getting.

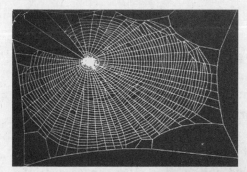

A normal orb web.

A normal orb web made by a spider on caffeine.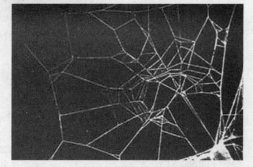

The impact of a drug "dose" is based on the child's weight. A can of soda for you is not the same as a can of soda for your child. A 12-ounce can of Coke has 35 milligrams of caffeine (Diet Coke has 45). If you put 35 milligrams of caffeine into a body that weighs 180 pounds, it diffuses a whole lot more than if you put it into a body that weighs 40 or 60 pounds. Basically, the same size can of soda has three times more effect on your child than it does on you. Think about that spiderweb picture when you think about the dose impact on your child.

As you think about caffeine, remember that it is found not just in coffee and soda. Here is a chart, based on information from the Center for Science in the Public Interest, that gives you a sense of the pervasiveness of caffeine in popular foods and drinks. I have included some things like Starbucks drinks because I have noticed so many children now consuming their specialty drinks like Frappucinos. As you look at this list, you may be confused by the differences in the caffeine content of the coffee and espresso drinks. Espresso has about 35 milligrams of caffeine in one ounce. Sixteen ounces of espresso would thus have about 560 milligrams of caffeine, or about twice the kick of regular brewed coffee. But most espresso drinks include just an ounce or two. You will note that Starbucks regular coffee has a very high octane that is about the same as espresso.

Product	Serving Size	Milligrams of Caffeine
Coffee, brewed	16 oz.	270
Starbucks Coffee, Grande	16 oz.	550
Starbucks Espresso	1 shot, 1 oz.	35
Starbucks Caffé Americano, tall, single shot	12 oz.	35
Starbucks Coffee, tall	12 oz.	375
Starbucks Caffé Mocha, tall	12 oz.	35
Tea, leaf or bag	8 oz.	50
7-Eleven Big Gulp	64 oz.	190
Cola	12 oz.	35
Mountain Dew	12 oz.	55
Diet Coke	12 oz.	45
Mello Yello	12 oz.	51
A & W Creme Soda	12 oz.	29
Dr Pepper	12 oz.	41
Sun Drop Regular	12 oz.	63
Sun Drop Diet	12 oz.	69

Product	Serving Size	Milligrams of Caffeine
Sunkist Orange Soda	12 oz.	41
Pepsi	12 oz.	38
Pepsi One	12 oz.	55
Royal Crown Cola	12 oz.	43
Royal Crown Edge	12 oz.	70
Snapple Iced Tea (all varieties)	16 oz.	48
Arizona Iced Tea	16 oz.	15–30
Java Water	½ liter	125
Juiced	10 oz.	60
Häagen-Dazs Coffee Ice Cream	1 c.	58
Dannon Coffee Yogurt	8 oz.	45
Hershey Special Dark Chocolate	1 bar, 1.5 oz.	31
NoDoz, maximum strength, or Vivarin	1	200

As you look at this chart, you can begin to see that, yes, caffeine drinks and foods can have a real impact on your child. If caffeine is a drug that lasts 3–7 hours in an adult, it is reasonable to assume that your child will experience drug withdrawal at the earlier end of that scale. So you may have a child in caffeine withdrawal who is edgy, irritable, cranky, and with a headache. So he can't sit still and is whining. You think he is· a bad boy. He gets the message he is a bad boy and begins to think of himself that way. And what is really happening is drug withdrawal, *not* being a bad boy.

I strongly encourage parents to get their children off of caffeine before dealing with the issue of sugar in sodas. But do not stop it abruptly. Going off of caffeine should be done through what I call a taper process, cutting down over time. Start by knowing the current level of caffeine each child is having. Use the same process you have been using all along. Do this *with* your child. Calculate the current level of caffeine intake, and then make a plan with your child to cut down. Replace the soda that has caffeine in it with soda that does not. I recommend cutting down on one-quarter of the total caffeine at a time, so getting off of it will take four weeks. Use this caffeine content list to make sure the alternate drinks you choose are caffeine free. I was surprised to learn that many drinks I assumed had no caffeine were spiked.

Liquid Candy

After you have done the caffeine part of step three, you will tackle the sugar aspect of it. Soda is the biggest source of refined sugar in the American diet. A typical teenage boy has 34 teaspoons of sugar a day, almost half of it coming from soda. Now that is a pretty scary statistic, yes? I am sharing this number so you can understand that your children's soda intake is *not* about your parenting. Your children are bombarded with the message to drink soda from everywhere. The task of getting the soda out of their diets is a tall order. Neither you nor your children are going to be able to "just say no" to soda in a flash.

Let me give you some tools that may help you help your child internalize why soda is such a bad alternative. Remember the spiderwebs? We saw that spiders on caffeine have a hard time organizing their webs. One particular web image, also produced by Peter Witt, is really scary. This spider was given dexamphetamine and sucrose. Putting speed and sugar together created the most disorganized web of all the drugs Witt studied. I thought about this and realized that caffeine and sugar are the two major ingredients in cola drinks. I wondered if they would be causing this kind of change in a child's brain. Let's say your ten-year-old son drinks a 20-ounce bottle of Pepsi at lunchtime. He weighs less than an adult, so it will have a much bigger effect on him than it might on you. And let's say he has been diag- nosed as having ADD. He

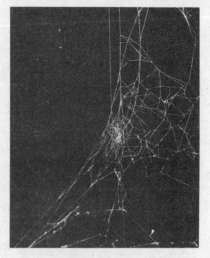

An orb web made by a spider given dexamphetamine and sucrose.

can't sit still and can't organize his thoughts. You are told to put him on Ritalin. The drug blasts his brain into being quiet. But the ADD is caused by the caffeine and sugar in the colas he is drinking. Wouldn't it be better to go to the cause rather than simply add another drug to mask his imbalance?

Let's create a striking alternative—*healing* the imbalance at its source. Not medicating it, not doing something to get rid of the symptoms, but actually fixing the problem. Granted, this approach is way harder than giving your child a pill. It requires time and involvement. It requires paying attention and negotiating, adjusting and dialoguing, but my hunch is you are ready for something different because you bought *Little Sugar Addicts*. I believe you are willing to do whatever it takes to get your child back. Step three is simple, but it is *not* easy.

*Tonight we were invited to a spur-of-the-moment picnic.
Our friends asked us to bring dessert. Eddie took the call
and reminded them we don't do dessert. Yippee! That part
felt nice. We did bring some fruit. Before leaving I talked
to the girls and asked them to make healthy food choices so
they wouldn't be cranky tonight or tomorrow. I reminded
them that there were bound to be lots of choices that
wouldn't be in their best interest. I then said, "and absolutely no soda." They sort of rolled their pretty little eyes
at me and said something like "Yeah, we know, Mom."*

*Lo and behold they made great dinner choices and
were running around with the kids playing games—
when I looked over to see them drinking from another
little girl's can of soda. What to do? I didn't want to embarrass them or make a big deal out of it. But I wanted
them to stop immediately so we wouldn't have to pay the
price later on. I decided to watch. Kayla took a drink
and put the can down. Lindsey took a drink, walked
away, then turned back around and went back to the
can. I could see her little addict self at work. One drink
was not enough.*

*I just nonchalantly went over and said in a clear,
calm voice, "No more soda, girls." The look on their
faces was kind of like a deer in the headlights. They gave
me the "Geez, Mom, we only had a couple of sips" line.
I just reminded them it was off limits. I didn't want to
pay the price of a can of soda later.*

*Hooray for me. No ambivalence. No charge, clear
and calm.*

Gail

You may start off being firm and saying "I am not going
to buy any more soda. We will drink water and juice now."

But your child will go to school where there are twenty vending machines all loaded up for him. So that infamous buy-in from your child becomes even more crucial when we get to the soda part. If you can help your children really buy in on a core level, you will get their compliance. Talk to them about neural disorganization. Many children will laugh and relate to this as a "brain fart." Copy the pictures of the spiderwebs from the book. Put them up on the refrigerator. Make extra copies. Send them to school. Have your children color them. Talk about the fact that you want the good web in your child's brain. Have them draw a web picture that shows what they think their brains look like.

Tell your child that going off even noncaffeine soda is the next piece of the healing puzzle. Here are the steps in the process. You and your kids can sort out a timetable.

- Stop using drinks that have caffeine in them. Work on doing this over four weeks so that no one goes into a withdrawal crisis.
- Shift from soda to juice. Ounce for ounce juice has the same amount of sugar as soda, so your child won't feel the sugar detox all at once. Once you do the conversion, then start diluting the juice. Many parents use sparkling water. A fizzy juice-water drink actually is very tasty, and kids really get the process. Start by replacing a quarter of the juice with water. Add more water each week until the kids complain. Then wait for two weeks and dilute more. Being sneaky works. If you go slowly, their tastebuds adjust and will be fine with a less intense juice taste. It doesn't really matter what juice you give them. Most of them are about the same sugar intensity. Stick with whole juice, and stay away from those that have high-

fructose corn syrup added. Some parents get real juice concentrate and use that with sparkling water.

- Offer milk rather than soda at meals. If your children prefer chocolate milk, use it to start with and then dilute it with white milk just as you do with the juices. Milk provides the calcium that growing bones need.
- Drink water, water, water, water. Make water the gold standard in your house.

This process will take a couple of months. Your children may really connect to the images of the spiderwebs. Somehow those pictures seem to really get to kids. Seeing an image makes it real.

Stress the water; keep the focus on what they can have rather than what they can't have. When you go to the ballgame or out for pizza, buy bottled water. Keep water in your car, and put water bottles in their backpacks. Make drinking water a habit. You can purchase bottled water in bulk at places like Costco and Sam's Club. Because of its popularity, you can buy bottled water nearly any place you buy soda.

What About Diet Soda?

What about using diet soda? It's not a good choice, for several reasons. The *taste* of sweet evokes beta-endorphin. Evoking beta-endorphin means keeping sugar cravings alive. Everything we are doing in the program is geared to reducing cravings and getting your kids off sugar. Diet products reinforce cravings and contradict where we are trying to go. And this is true of all alternative sweeteners, even the ones like stevia that do not affect blood sugar levels.

Besides evoking beta-endorphin, aspartame is especially not a good alternative for your children. Aspartame is made from three different things: aspartic acid, methyl alcohol, and phenylalanine. When the body tries to handle the methyl alcohol, it breaks it down into formaldehyde. How scary is that? I told several twelve-year-old boys about Diet Coke creating embalming fluid (formaldehyde), and they were truly upset. They stopped drinking diet soda that day. If you meet kids where they are, you will get results.

Phenylalanine is an amino acid with a very sweet taste. It is a precursor to dopamine, the brain chemical that gives you a feeling of being up and alert. It is the neurochemical that is targeted by cocaine and amphetamine. It creates a sense of brightness and competence. Putting more of the precursor in the blood sets up greater availability for the factory to make more. Because of this dopamine "pushing" effect, I believe that aspartame is highly addictive, particularly in sugar sensitive people. Regular use of it creates a physical dependence. And physical dependence means withdrawal on discontinuance.

Some years ago, despite my growing sense of unease about aspartame, I continued to drink diet soda. It seemed harmless enough and provided a nice alternative if I wanted to have something to drink with lunch. And yes, I know that this kind of rationalization is the hallmark of an addictive personality. At one point I decided to quit using it. On the third day after I stopped, I woke up feeling really, really depressed. I felt as if I could not move my arms and that my brain was in a dark hole. This truly startled me since I am not a depressive sort of person. I was baffled by the darkness I felt until I remembered that I had stopped using diet soda. I wondered if there was a connection. I went and got a can of diet soda, and within five minutes of drinking it I felt just fine. In fact, I felt clear, relaxed, and ready for the world. This got my attention in a big way. I tried this experiment several times, and the result was the same every time.

I started asking members of our community if anyone felt they were hooked on diet soda. People from everywhere in the community wanted to talk about it. I heard stories about how dependent they felt on it, how driven to use it, and how difficult to get off it. About this same time I was talking with a thirteen-year-old boy and told him I felt he was ready to go off of sugar. We had been talking for a while, and this seemed like the logical next step as he had cut his sugar intake and was ready for the next challenge.

Two days later his mother reported to me that he was crawling through the day and felt like death warmed over. He was acting like a bear, and she was concerned. It made no sense to me because I knew what his sugar intake had been. The reaction seemed truly disproportionate. Then his mother told me that he was a diet soda junkie and had decided to quit that as well. No wonder he was in such big trouble. Always factor this variable in as you plan for change with your children. Do not have them go off of diet soda cold turkey. Taper, then stop.

Be Kind and Taper

Many sugar addicts think the idea of tapering off is silly. They feel terrible and want to get rid of the offending drug as soon as possible, be it sugar, caffeine, or aspartame. They figure if they are going to face feeling bad, they might as well just feel *really* bad and get it over with, bite the bullet, feel horrible for a few days, and be done with it. This belief is indicative of addictive thinking—the magic cure, no work, and lots of drama.

From a physiological point of view, this is absolutely the worst possible way to make change. Your body and your brain cannot catch up to your enthusiasm. Your system is in shock rather than in healing mode. The first weeks of detox are spent recuperating from the shock rather than building biochemical restoration. If you do a taper, at the end of four weeks you will have the same outcome on the outside, but with a body that has spent four weeks healing rather than trying to recuperate from shock. On the outside you might look the same as someone who goes "cold turkey," but on the inside there is no comparison.

This is even truer for children. You want to minimize the shock effect as much as possible. As children's bodies are growing, their brains are continuing to develop, and a host of new cells are constantly being created. This is what growth is about. You want to maximize stability and steadiness to help support the changes your child is going through. You want your child's developmental energy to be going toward making sense of the world rather than compensating for a biochemical disturbance.

Follow the steps I have outlined in this chapter slowly and in order. Each step is a refinement in your child's relationship to sugar. Each step builds on the one before it. Each incremental shift in food is intentional and is done to maximize the impact of the whole healing. In this step, you are adding in snacks and taking out soda. Nothing more.

6

Step Four:
Lunch and Dinner

Before we talk about what to put in the other two meals of the day, let me share a little about lunch and dinner for children. The most important rule is *eating on time*. Most sugar sensitive parents have trouble providing regular meals on time. You get distracted or involved or busy, and you "forget" that it is already 11:30 and your child needs to eat lunch soon. You figure the snack will tide her over and she will be fine. You know that you can push yourself a little more and just finish up. That may be true for your grown-up body; it is not true for your child.

So step four means paying attention to time. I know, you thought I was going to say you have to pay attention to food. Yep, that, too. But first let's do time. Children really cannot go more than about three hours without eating. Your job as a parent is to make sure they have food on time. Most parents think the contents of meals are the most crucial. They get very motivated and think about what to feed their children and don't really factor in *when*. The more I talk with sugar sensitive parents, the more aware I have become about the "when" factor.

Lunch

Let's start with the children who eat at home with you (or a caregiver). These will be little ones who are not in day-care or are with you throughout the weekend and of course in the evening. Do a quick review, and see if time is an issue for you. What are your typical routines? Do you even know when your children eat lunch? Start with what is easiest in making a time change. It may be week-ends, or it may be your weekday routine. Take a week and see if you can get all the lunchtimes you have con-trol over within the same thirty-minute period every day. Just try this first step, and work with your children on it. Get a sense of what parts of your family's routine sup-port this goal and what messes up your plan. Just as we have seen all along, knowing what gets in the way will give you choices about what you need to do to make this successful.

Marty always gets in trouble on Saturday. She takes her three kids out to do Saturday errands. She has "just one more thing" to do and pushes the time edge until her kids are falling off the cliff. One boy starts getting wild at three and a half hours. The other starts to whine at three hours. Her daughter gets pale and quiet after two hours.

Suzanne is fine with her kids on the weekend but has a terrible time during the week. She works out of her home and is frequently on the phone. Eleven becomes 12:30 in a flash. She has sweet kids; they are very cooperative and don't whine or create a problem. She just didn't notice that they got pale and lay down on the couch at 11:30. She just thought they were being good.

Many parents really have to work on this one. Be kind and gentle with yourself. Talk with your children and see if you all can identify ways to have everyone help remember lunchtime. Set an alarm clock. Give the five-year-old a digital watch so she can come remind you. Write out a meal schedule (or let the young ones do it), and put it on the refrigerator. If everyone goes off to school, plan for the weekend. Talk about lunch at breakfast time. What are the plans? Where? When? And then of course, what?

Lunch needs to have the same amount of protein as breakfast. By now, you and your kids know the protein drill. Sit down with them and talk about lunch options. Be very specific. If they have fast-food choices at school, have *them* sort out which ones will work. They may discover that they need a supplemental protein package. Talk with them about what will work.

Here is a list of fast-food alternatives that our community parents came up with. Many of these work well for lunch. Have your children add to it, and then bring their new discoveries online to share with the other kids at www.radiantkids.com.

- Greek souvlaki wrap
- Wendy's burger with double meat
- Wendy's baked potato with a burger broken up and added to the chili topping
- Subway sandwich with extra meat and cheese
- nuts and diluted apple juice

- deli meat wrapped around a cheese stick
- foil-packed tuna and mayo with crackers
- beef jerky
- Taco Bell taco, with extra meat and cheese
- hard-boiled egg
- dehydrated soup in a cup with add-your-own chicken
- soup and a salad bar salad topped with extra chicken
- large pretzel and string cheese
- nachos with cheese and chili
- peanut butter and sliced banana on crackers
- egg salad in a Styrofoam cup eaten with Fritos
- hot dog topped with cheese
- "rice bowl" with extra meat and less rice

Now, not all these choices are "ideal" nutritionally, but they are options when you and your kids are on the go, and they are way better than chips and Coke. Remember we are doing baby steps. And an interesting thing often happens when children start eating "real" food. They want more, and they want better. They may come back to you and say "Mom, can't you make something better?" This is a wonderful opportunity for you to suggest that *they* do it with you. Many kids love to cook. Invite them to help you. Check out the recipes in the back of this book. Things like Easy Does It Pizza (see page 226) and Chicken Drummettes (see page 227) are very easy to make and make great lunches. Macaroni and Cheese Pie (see page 231) and tomato soup make a great lunch.

If you don't cook, think about finding a cooking class for children. Ask the Y, and check the adult education options in your community. If you don't find anything, talk to those organizations about starting one. Talk to your child's teacher about including a unit on cooking. Get your own children a set of smaller utensils and pots, and teach them. My daughter got a set of real miniature mixers for her three-year-old. He loves mixing things and then cooking them. I taught my eight-year-old grandson how to use a sharp paring knife. His mother was skittish; he was thrilled with the new skill and now loves cutting vegetables. When he cuts them, they are "his," and he wants to eat them. Learning skills enhances buy-in. If you or your kids pack your own lunch, think about using the "wraps, stacks, and layers" approach.

Wraps, Stacks, and Layers

Tortillas can be a very versatile part of your program—you can stuff and wrap them, stack them, roll them, layer them, broil them, bake them, grill them. Think of a tortilla as a blank canvas upon which you can paint any cuisine that strikes your fancy. Avoid the traditional white flour tortillas, and look for tortillas made with whole grains. Refined white flour seems to act very much like sugar in many sugar sensitive children. I will talk more about "browning" your family in step five, but for now you can experiment with the whole wheat, blue corn, white corn, spelt, and oat bran tortillas that you can purchase in many supermarkets and natural food stores. If you have a hard time finding nonwhite alternatives, try the recipes for Cornbread Crepes (see page 220) or Kathleen's Baking Mix Wraps (see page 213). Practice with whole grain and bean flours to make your own pancake-type tortilla. There are no rules in what you make, so feel free to experiment to your heart's content.

Wraps can be served hot or cold. Here are some filling options. I know that some of them may seem sophisticated for your kids, but don't make assumptions. Ask them.

- grilled chicken, mayo, lettuce, tomato, and onion
- scrambled eggs, potatoes, chili, cheese, and beans
- chicken salad with grapes and walnuts (make your own from leftovers, or buy it at the deli)
- grilled salmon and roasted red pepper dressing
- roasted veggies with shrimp/chicken/pork
- stir-fry veggies with shrimp/chicken/pork
- sandwich meats and cheeses piled high
- Sloppy Joes made from ground hamburger or turkey and Sloppy Joe Mix
- Navajo Taco—ground beef, beans, lettuce, onion, tomato, and salsa
- peanut butter and apples and raisins
- planned-over meat loaf, cheese, and sliced tomato
- tuna salad with apples
- egg salad with roasted dry onion flakes and tomatoes

Stacks are made by piling tortillas high with ingredients and broiling. Try these:

- pizza of tomato sauce, cheese, veggies, and meats
- pizza with sausage and four kinds of cheeses (mozzarella, cheddar, jack, havarti)
- pizza with ham and unsweetened canned pineapple

Layers can be made by alternating tortillas and filling. Start with a layer of tortillas, then a layer of filling, then another layer of tortillas, another layer of filling, and a

final layer of tortillas on top. Many of us sprinkle shredded mozzarella cheese on top. Bake some for today's
meal, and refrigerate the rest:

- lasagna (corn tortillas, tomato sauce, hamburger,
  cheddar cheese and whatever spices your family will
  like)
- green chili chicken or seafood enchiladas
- red chili beef enchiladas
- pesto, sun-dried tomato, and chicken and cheese

Quesadillas are another variation on a wrap. Split and
stuff the tortilla, fill, and broil. Then cut in quarters. Use:

- grilled chicken strips, mashed pinto beans, and Mon-
  terey jack cheese
- mashed black beans, grilled green peppers, rice, and
  cheddar cheese
- crumbled sausage, sliced tomato and onions, and
  shredded mozzarella cheese
- scrambled eggs, ham, and sliced Swiss cheese
- sausage-and-egg-bake planned-overs (see page 225)

Now, I know you are muttering, "Kathleen! Pesto! With
my eight-year-old!" But I speak from experience. When
you turn kids loose in the kitchen, sometimes they get really excited about things you would never dream of. If you
have lots of basil in your garden, let your kids make pesto,
or try a prepared pesto from a place like Trader Joe's or
Whole Foods Market. And be sure to check the recipes in
this book. Many of them are very kid friendly and suitable
for your children to make themselves.

The other solid way to do lunch is with planned-overs. When you make dinner, make extra. Sit down with your children and outline their favorite dinners. Put that list up where everyone can see it. Think ahead and plan for the days when lunch that has been made from leftover dinner will work. Remember that you can make extra food at dinnertime with the specific idea of having enough left for the next day's lunch.

Remember that lunch will come again. And even if you are incredibly tired and you cannot imagine adding one more chore like planning lunch to your morning tasks, know that the longer you do breakfast well and within an hour, the easier lunch becomes.

Lunch at school is more of a dilemma. The kids in our community have told me that bringing lunch from home is not cool. If this is true for your children, then you will need to do some more negotiating. Sit down with your children and talk about what the lunch options are. The starting point is actually "eating" something, since many kids choose chips and soda for lunch. If the school uses fast-food vendors, then help your children make choices among what is being offered. A submarine sandwich from Subway is better than chips and soda. A hamburger with a stuffed baked potato is a fine alternative. Pizza is better than nothing. Get your kids involved. By now they have a sense of the drill and can be your best ally in sorting out the day-to-day specifics of lunch.

A fast-food tutorial can be fun for all of you. Back to the drawing board. Identify all the fast-food places your children love (or have available at lunchtime). Go online, and do a Google search for nutrient analysis of fast foods. Let your children sort out how much protein is in a Quarter

Pounder or Chicken McNuggets. Do not be a purist. This is about making the best choices you can. Make up a three-by-five card of choices that suit you and your kids, and put one on your car visor with a rubber band so you always have it with you. Have your kids make one for each of them and keep it in their backpack. When you or the kids are hungry, the list of best choices is hard to remember. You will run into the gas station and draw a blank on what you can eat and then grab a candy bar.

As you start this process, you may feel that there is no way your children will ever be able to do something differently, no way they could say "not for me" when all their friends are having soda and sweets. They won't right away. But over time, if they buy in, they will. I listen to the kids on the kids' group in our community talking about lunches at school. The same kids who two years ago did not want to hear any of this are now sharing with one another ideas for lunches brought from home, healthy, solid lunches packed with protein and healthy breads. They are not superkids, they are eight- and eleven- and thirteen-year-olds who get the program on a personal level. And even more surprising, they see how awful most of the school choices are. They bring up issues with teachers about not serving cupcakes and they ask teachers to tell the principal to get good foods in the cafeteria. I am not kidding. These are the very kids who used to say, "Well, Daddy lets me have two sodas, so I'm going to have them with my lunch."

Over time you may find that you and your kids plan for being out and take food with you. Most of our parents now plan ahead and have little coolers in the car stocked with cheese, hard-boiled eggs, sugar-free jerky, crackers, apple juice, V-8 juice, and water. They carry foil packs of tuna or chicken. They put packs of dehydrated cheese snacks from our online store in the glove compartment.

Dinner

Just as you did with lunch, do your research plan first. What variables affect dinner in your house? Do both parents work? What time does everyone get in? How much time do you have between getting home and eating? Are you all on different schedules? Do you all eat together? Do you get carry-out food four times a week? Do you eat in front of the TV? Do you look forward to dinner? Is dinner peaceful or chaotic? Answering these questions is the same deal as with each of our fact-finding missions: no judgment, just the data. This is crucial because you are going to start from where you are, not from where you wish you were.

Okay, so the first task once again is **time**. If your spouse doesn't get home till 7:30, you will need to give the kids dinner earlier. They cannot wait that long. Most children really need to eat no later than six, especially if lunch was six hours earlier. Even a healthy snack won't hold them much longer into the evening. I suspect that for many of you dinner in the past has been very stressful. The kids are tired and cranky and bicker with one another or stand by you and whine while you are trying to clear your brain enough to think what to make for dinner. Adding the snacks in will make a huge difference. Blood sugar levels will not be falling, and your kids can cope while waiting for dinner.

I am a great believer in creating some quiet time for

yourself while you catch your breath and then fix the meal. Put on the TV or a video if you need to, and let the kids switch gears as well. Don't be afraid to use the TV as a tool for psychic space. You need realistic support to make a long-term change, and this includes getting your own quiet time. If you do not watch TV in your house, make sure your kids have a stash of crayons, markers, and other art supplies, fresh puzzles and games, or new books from the library. You know your own children. Plan for what will give *you* downtime.

Picky Eaters

Okay, so what if you have picky eaters, or children who like different things? Once again we are going to start with where your family is and then plan to move to where you would like your family to be. Sugar sensitive children who are still biochemically imbalanced will eat what they have to in order to get to dessert at the end of dinner. Often meals are one big conversation about "How much do I have to eat" to get the cake. Rather than continuing a power game on this topic, you are going to shift a few rules, one at a time. The first is: everyone has to have the right amount of protein. By now, older kids will know how to get enough. Let them figure out what they have to eat. Have them tell you the answer to that question. If they have the meal, serve dessert if you generally do that. Even though you have not yet moved to a sugar-free household, you can start to make program-friendly desserts. Check the recipe section for some yummy alternatives like Blueberry Cream Parfait (see page 252) and Baked Apples with Walnut Sauce (see page 245). The Apple Pie with Cheddar Crust (see page 248) is so yummy that your family will ask for it over and over. Apple Pear Compote (see page 240) is a great dessert to use for company.

As you start working with dinner, you might find that you get interested in trying some new dishes. As your own chemistry settles, you may feel like cooking. I have included a recipe for Kathleen's Baking Mix (see page 213) in the recipe section. It is a mix that I use to make the things I used to make with a standard white flour mix. It is whole grain and works perfectly for my program. I even use it to make Quickie Oven-Fried Chicken (see page 229). Choose the foods that you like to make and that your family likes to eat. Use dinner as a time for the whole family to connect. Create the time and space to make dinner an event.

Don't forget vegetables. Ah, veggies, the thing that so many parents forget. If your vegetable skills lie pretty much with serving peas and corn, be bold and try some new ways to make vegetables. Get the kids to help. Try the Carrot Apple Bake (see page 234) or Cranberry-Glazed Acorn Squash (see page 235). I recently bought a new variety of squash because it was so pretty. I couldn't even find the name of the variety. But when I was making a roasted chicken, I put that squash in the oven along with the chicken. When I took the chicken out, the squash was soft and smelled wonderful. I cut it open, scooped out the seeds, and put some butter and cinnamon on it. It was just super! Try making Roasted Garlic Mashed Potatoes (see page 237). Make extra, and then use the leftovers to make potato pancakes the next morning.

Given the work you have already been doing with your kids on breakfast and lunch, dinner should be pretty straightforward. But it may not be. You may have some residual patterns that you need to work through. I want to talk about some of these because I think it is hard for parents to see the forest for the trees when they are in the middle of it. You may have children who don't eat, or who are picky eaters and eat only one thing. You may have screamers or stonewallers who will sit in a power struggle for two hours over the peas. You are going to step out of old patterns. These things may naturally change just by changing your style from "You have to eat what I say" to "Let's eat what works for you." But it may not. Your job is to remember that you are the boss. Even if your little five-year-old can outsit you anytime over the peas. The reality is you know more about this situation, and you understand what is at stake in terms of your child's well-being. In this case, if peas aren't working, don't serve peas! Above all, don't engage in a power struggle. Have the children tell you what will work. If they like different things, have them sort out how to handle that. Try giving them the parameters and allowing them to make the choices inside them. If you tell them you won't serve peas, ask for something in return. What will work? Engage them in the process. You don't want to turn into a short-order cook if you are dealing with more than one child, but you could provide a "dinner bar" like the breakfast bar with different proteins and veggies. It's okay to let them have a peanut butter sandwich if they hate meat loaf. Have them work out the protein amount they need, tell them what you are fixing, and then have them come up with a solution.

Hard-core Stonewallers

If you do all this and you still get a child refusing to eat, simply excuse them from the table and allow them to go to another room, but explain they can have no TV, no computer, and no GameBoy while the rest of the family is still eating. Explain that you don't want Grumpy to be a part of dinner. And do not, *do not* give in about having something later. You may be thinking, "But Kathleen, their blood sugar is tumbling. You said to be vigilant about *that!*" True, but it is fine to take a few nights to shift old patterns. Bear in mind, your child will have breakfast in the morning. You are simply going to take the charge out of the "fight." Fighting raises beta-endorphin levels. If you take away the benefit of fighting, you significantly alter the pattern. If your child chooses to skip a meal, you can let it go. And if your approach remains consistent, she'll quickly eat according to the new ground rules, and eventually she will adapt. Hang in there.

The key here is that you do not want to fight over anything that has to do with food. As I have said to you before, you do not have to fight because **you are the boss**. You are the parent trying to do what is best for your child. You may have lost sight of that because little sugar addicts can be pretty feisty, and you may have given in because you were just too tired to go at it again. But breakfast is transforming you. Now you will stay calm and have a sense of humor and say, "We are not fighting about dinner. If you don't like what we are doing, you may leave the room." You see, first you are going to set the ground rules about how you do dinner; then you will set ground rules about the contents of dinner. If you are reading this before you have actually made the breakfast and lunch changes, this process may feel a little scary. It would be if you were just forging ahead and doing it. But you are not. You are coming to it after a lot of change you have already made. If you have been following the steps in the previous chapters, your children will have a context for the dinner ground rules.

Support from Other Adults in Your Family

There is one other critical piece in the equation: whether or not your spouse, partner, or other adult in your home supports your efforts. You will need to talk about dinnertime before you make this change. All adults have to be on board about it. If you say, "Okay, you may leave the table now," and Daddy or Grandma pipes up, "Absolutely not, you *will* finish your peas," then all your groundwork will go down the tubes. Get all the grown-ups on board beforehand. Talk through the rationale of this one. Provide context. Create the buy-in so all of you are in agreement about where you want to get to and how to do it. If you have never done this, or have never done this about food, take the time to raise these issues with the other adults before you take action with the kids. If you need to bide your time while you come to a mutual adult understanding, do so.

Fast Foods

Many parents rely on take-out foods during the week. Everyone is tired and hungry after school and work, and cooking is not an option. What to do? I asked our community parents what they do and was really startled by the answers they gave. A large majority of those who had been doing the program for more than a year laughed and said, "I get a roasted chicken from the deli or grocery store, make nuked potatoes [in the microwave], and make frozen veggies." Now, I swear they had not talked with one another about this before we had that chat. It seemed to be an organic and logical solution. The newer parents talked about going to Wendy's and getting hamburgers and baked potatoes, or getting Chinese take-out with extra meat and less rice, or getting pizza with salad and added meat and cheese. The list on pages 112–13 also includes options for dinner in a rush.

Working the Plan on a Budget

Some of you may be working with a limited budget, and when you think about the impact on your grocery budget of all this "good" food, you get overwhelmed. You know you can't afford "fancy foods" and the prices in health foods store are beyond your means. You groan because you are struggling to make ends meet, and yet you are being told to up the protein in your family's diet.

The secret to making change is just like the program: you do it in baby steps, and you plan carefully. Let's start with the proteins. They don't have to be fancy. Pinto beans or peanut butter are great. Tuna, eggs, and chicken all work. It doesn't need to be gourmet stuffed chicken breast; thighs on sale are fine. Don't spook yourself. You are already skilled at stretching a dollar. What you are going to do is make artful trades. For example, if you buy plain oatmeal instead of sugared cereals and spend the difference on extra tuna, you will be on your way. How much have you been spending on sugary sodas, cookies, and other junk foods? Fifteen or twenty dollars a week, maybe? You can buy an awful lot of chicken thighs or pinto beans for that amount.

If money has been an issue for you, I suspect you are

already very skilled and creative when you go to the store. You may know how to buy inexpensive food, but now it is time to shift your thinking on what you buy. Let's say you have been eating Kraft Macaroni and Cheese three nights a week. It doesn't offer much nutrition, but it fills you up without costing a lot. So now you buy whole wheat macaroni in bulk and use cheddar cheese and canned tuna. It's the same basic meal but a thousand times better for you, and per serving, it will be cheaper than the brand-name mac and cheese.

You may choose to make your own whole wheat tortillas or pancakes, then fill them with canned or homemade beans, cheese, and vegetables. It's cheaper to serve oatmeal and eggs than Pop-Tarts. Lentil soup and brown rice is about as good a meal as you can get, and it is way easier on your wallet than fast food. And dry milk is a great protein source and staple to have on hand. Add it to all sorts of things. When I suggest making a shake in the morning, you can make the very same thing using dry milk powder, oatmeal, and ripe bananas.

We asked some of the members of our community what changes they made when they were on a limited budget. Here are the things they shared:

- "I buy items in bulk by going in with my friends and shopping at Sam's Club. We started planning together sort of as a game. Now it's fun. We kinda have our own little buying club."
- "I buy items on sale and stock up. I know the basic things I use and plan for when the sales come up. I think the planning thing is the biggest change. Of course the longer I'm doing the program, the less helpless I feel about having such a limited budget."

- "I buy fruits and vegetables that are in season. My store has a place for bruised or cut vegetables and fruits, and I get them and just cut out the damage. I have talked with the produce guy, and he told me the best day to find things. In fact, he loves to help me get the good stuff."

- "I planted my own tomatoes and veggies. My kids helped. We had fun, and they *loved* eating from their own garden. They used to turn their noses up at vegetables. But when they are their own vegetables, they rub 'em and scrub 'em."

- "I shop online for vitamins/protein powders and watch for the sales. I was surprised at how much cheaper things were."

- "I started to make my own whole grain bread. My kids love it so much, they haven't even noticed it's brown. We use it for peanut butter sandwiches for breakfast. They have that and a glass of milk, and it seems to work really well for them."

- "I grew up on beans and rice and corn and tomatoes from the garden. Funny, we were never sick. I went away from this as I got older. But I am trying it out. My brain remembers what to do. I am making brown rice instead of white. My family is actually pleased. We even made some homemade tortillas, and they were great!"

- "I get food stamps and usually just roam the aisles deciding. Last time I actually made a plan before I went. I left the kids at home so they wouldn't ask for things. I ate before I went. What a difference it made. I spent the same amount of money but got totally different things. I am even thinking about using my commodity foods in a different way."

- "I made this *huge* pot of lentil stew with ham hocks. It smelled so good, my kids are asking for it every week. Then I got brave. We usually have franks and beans on Saturday night. Last week, I *made* the beans and made some brown bread. Surprised even me!"

- "When we looked at what we were spending for Cokes, beer, and chips, it stunned both my kids and me. Now we buy some more protein, get better bread stuff, and spend some on videos. It is a nice trade."

Working the Plan with Time Constraints

Money may not be the issue for some of you, but time is a problem. Doing this program involves taking time to think, time to talk, time to shop, and time to cook, and you are a busy parent juggling work, home, and life. What options are there for you?

Don't spook yourself. Yes, it takes time to talk with your kids and to achieve the buy-in. But talking with the kids is crucial, and you and I both know that this is a good thing. Doing the food is simply going to nudge you to do what you know is good. And surprisingly, as you do your own program, time will expand. Sugar sensitivity untreated makes for frantic and chaotic households. That will change, and you are going to be shocked at how much time you find.

Find people to help with food preparation. You might want to hire a personal chef to come in once a week to cook and leave yummy meals in the refrigerator for the week. You might find a teen who loves to cook and would be delighted not only to baby-sit but to cook with your children. Use the deli at stores like Whole Foods. The choices are awesome. A precooked chicken is a great start for your family meal. Ask your kids to help. Use the time to talk and cook.

The Pay-off

The pay-off from step four is huge. It may take some time, even months, to master lunch and dinner, but these changes are going to have an unexpected impact on your family. You are going to see that the picture is way bigger than sugar. Regular meals, with enough to eat, with solid protein and healthy carbohydrates, are going to cumulatively add up, and you will start to see big and positive changes.

7

Step Five:
"Browning" Your Family

We have talked some about the importance of having complex carbohydrates in your family's diet. Sugar sensitive children can react to refined carbohydrates as if they were sugars. Refined carbohydrates or "white things" have had the fiber taken out; chemically speaking, they are the "short necklace" carbohydrates, with fewer molecules in their makeup. These foods, among them white flour baked goods, look attractive but are broken down and digested very rapidly and can spike blood sugar. Unlike many popular weight-loss plans that espouse no or low carbohydrates, my plan recommends "slow" carbohydrates. Slow carbohydrates or "brown things" retain the part of the grain that has the most nutrition. They are high in fiber that takes longer for the body to digest. Slow carbohydrates are the molecule-packed chemical necklaces with lots and lots of "beads." The longer the necklace or molecular chain, the longer it takes to break down. And the resulting longer, or slower, digestion time means that brown things contribute to more stable blood sugar.

Here is a chart from *Potatoes Not Prozac* that will give you a sense of the relative "brown" value of many of the foods your family eats. I call it the carbohydrate continuum.

THE CARBOHYDRATE CONTINUUM

Alcohol	Simple Sugars	Simple Starch	Complex Starches	Complex Starches	Wood Starches
beer wine	glucose sucrose fructose white sugar honey corn syrup all the others	"white things" white flour products white rice pasta	"brown things" whole grains beans potatoes roots	"green things" broccoli green vege- tables "yellow things" squash yellow vege- tables	not digestible (by humans)

Your body eventually breaks all carbohydrates down to glucose. How quickly it can do this depends on how complex the food is. The foods on the left of the Carbohydrate Continuum are very simple, with only a few molecules. They are absorbed rapidly. The foods on the right are very complex and require the body to work hard to break them down. This takes a long time and means that you will not get a sugar "high" from broccoli!

There are three main areas in your family's food program that will need browning: cereal, bread, and pasta products. The level of fiber in the product provides information about how brown the product is. More fiber means browner. For example, one slice of white bread has 12 grams of carbohydrate and no fiber, while one slice of whole grain bread (Arnold Bran'nola) has 17.5 grams of carbohydrate and 2.9 grams of fiber.

Your local natural foods store will have some very heavy, very brown bread, but realistically, you will not want to get this bread for your children. It is what I call "scary" bread and is the last thing you want to buy. Your children would go on strike if you offered it to them. But there are lots and lots of choices in between. The key is to find whole grain bread that is so yummy, your kids will actually prefer it over the white stuff. Let them choose from different options. As you have learned by now, if they choose, they will at least be willing to try. Read labels and look for breads with higher fiber.

The Whole Foods Market supermarket chain has a kind of bread called Seeduction that is very wholesome. It is made with whole grain flours and has a fair amount of molasses in it, so it tastes sweet. As sugars go, molasses is nutritious and will buffer the switch to browner bread. And until you go to step six, where you start taking the sugars out, it is fine to have bread with molasses in it. In fact, with your children, it may be fine even then.

Here is how I know about this particular bread and its molasses content. Last year several of my volunteers came out to help with a health fair. I knew the food at the fairground would be, shall we say, limited and that fry bread and cola were not quite our best choices. I went to Whole Foods and got what looked like wonderful bread (I did not read the label), picked up sliced chicken, avocado, and tomatoes, and made some awesome sandwiches. We loved those sandwiches in a big way. We wanted more, for dinner and for breakfast. We sucked up those sandwiches. And we laughed and laughed because of course we *knew*!!

Anytime a food "calls" in a big way, it is triggering the old sugar addict brain.

The early transition to browning is about substitution. Use browner bread for white bread, and choose higher-fiber cereal instead of the sugared stuff. White things are everywhere. Pancakes, waffles, muffins, tortillas, bagels, pasta—all the things we love the most tend to be made with white flour. With the exception of foods like croissants and authentic French bread, nearly all whites can be converted to brown. Do this slowly. Do it a little at a time. Do not scare your family, but be firm.

Most people find the conversion from white pasta to whole grain pasta the hardest of the brownings. Whole wheat pasta has a strange texture. Some families love it, I hate it. Try getting pasta made from brown rice flour. It has a wonderful flavor that seems to go over much better than the heavier, grainy feel of whole wheat pasta, so your family may accept the switch more easily. Do the pasta change last, after your family is more accustomed to whole grains.

Let's take a look at some of the cereals your family may be using. This chart can give you a sense of how brown the cereal is. Look in the column that shows the percentage of fiber.

Cereal Name	Serving Size	Carb Grams	Sugar Grams	Percentage of Sugar	Fiber Grams	Percentage of Fiber
All-Bran Extra Fiber	½ cup	22	6.3	28%	14	6%
Cap'n Crunch	¾ cup	23.8	11.4	48%	.8	3%
Cheerios	1¼ cups	19.6	1.0	5%	2.0	10%
Corn Chex	1 cup	25	3.0	12%	1.1	4%

Cereal Name	Serving Size	Carb Grams	Sugar Grams	Percentage of Sugar	Fiber Grams	Percentage of Fiber
Count Chocula	1 cup	24	13.0	54%	0	0%
Fruity Marshmallow Krispies	1¼ cups	32	17.0	53%	0	0%
Grape-Nuts	¼ cup	23	3.4	15%	2.6	11%
Raisin Bran	¾ cup	31	13.0	38%	5	16%
Rice Krispies	1 cup	24.8	2.0	8%	0	0%
Special K	1⅓ cups	21.3	3.0	14%	0	0%
Shredded Wheat	1 biscuit	18.8	.1	0%	2.2	12%

It is sort of dramatic to see the comparisons, yes? This is a wonderful exercise you can do with your children. You can either go online or you can find a book by Jean Pennington called *Food Values of Portions Commonly Used*. This book is out of print but very valuable. It's considered the gold standard for nutritional information in book form. I like it because it's one of the few resources that includes sugar content. You might use it to have your kids calculate the cereals they eat and the breads your family chooses.

After you have experimented with alternative substitutions for white bread and white cereals, let's take a look at how you can use brown things in other places creatively. You have been looking at how to introduce products with a higher percentage of fiber (those that are browner). You can also try using whole wheat flour instead of refined white flour in the foods you make yourself. Many baking books say not to substitute whole grain for refined flour on a one-to-one basis because whole grains are much denser. Many recipes suggest a ratio of one part refined flour to a half part whole grain flour (1 : ½). For instance, if a recipe calls for two cups of white flour, you would use one cup white flour and a half cup of whole grain. This is a step in the right direction, but it also reflects the traditional viewpoint that refined is best. As you move from white things to brown things, you will want to leave the refined flour out entirely. Experiment with different flours to see the ones your family will tolerate best. I use a mixture of oat flour and brown rice flour.

Other Types of Flour

You can also experiment with using other types of flour than just whole wheat. The nonwheat flours on the market have special flavors and textures and so are fun to experiment with when you have some time and interest. Some sugar-free children are sensitive to wheat. You can watch to see if your child gets sleepy or cranky after having wheat. If so, changing to nonwheat alternatives may help his overall sense of well-being. I am wheat sensitive and so have looked for creative alternatives. You will see that Kathleen's Baking Mix in our recipe section (see page 213) is wheat free. *The Gluten-Free Gourmet Cooks Fast and Healthy* by Bette Hagman and Joseph A. Murray makes some substitution suggestions for replacing 1 cup of white flour:

- 1 cup whole wheat flour
- ⅞ cup rice flour
- ⅝ cup potato starch
- 1 cup corn flour
- 1 scant cup fine cornmeal

I am not a baker, so I enlisted a chef to help me experiment with white and wheat flour substitutions. We went through a good deal of trial and error and had a few disasters. Finally, we found a solution that worked every time. Replace 1 cup of wheat flour with ½ cup of oat flour and ½ cup of brown rice flour. The oats give body and the brown rice gives lightness. You will see this combination in many of the recipes in this book. It serves well in a wide range of things from pie crusts to cookies to baking mixes to quick breads. It also works for coating meats before browning and for thickening gravies. It is not foolproof— it makes a horrible angel food cake. "Play" with the combination and see what works for you.

Let's take a look at some of the alternative grains. As you learn to use them, first taste the grain alone to get a sense of its texture and taste, then try combining different types of grains in the same dish. Have your kids try each as you go.

Cooking Grains

Since preparing whole grains takes more time and effort than simply making five-minute rice, you might want to invest in a rice cooker. I got a little one at Wal-Mart for under ten dollars. They are so foolproof, even your young children can use them. You can prepare any of these grains in a rice cooker and serve them as a brown side dish, as you would rice or potatoes. When you first read this section, you may laugh at the idea of using these grains. You may think, "Oh Kathleen, there you go again! I am a working mom, I am tired when I get home. This stuff takes time. You have got to be kidding." Nope, I am not. Get that rice cooker. Put the grains on to cook when you walk in the door. Or be outrageous and have your kids help. They can start the cooker before you get home. I am asking you to think out of the box and try something you haven't done before. I have come to really love these grain alternatives, and I want you to share in that discovery. And your kids don't have to tell anyone they are eating something as strange as quinoa (pronounced *qeen wah*). It can be a family secret.

Now, don't just skip this section and go on to step six. Browning is fun! And new grains are a large part of browning. While a side dish of cooked whole grains can add to any meal, they can also provide lots of other options for your family's meals.

- Add several tablespoons of cooked grains to stews, soups, and vegetable salads.
- Mix leftover grains with beaten eggs to make "pancakes." I use a ½ cup cooked grain and add two eggs for one serving.
- Use a hot breakfast cereal with the addition of warm milk, chopped fresh seasonable fruits, and flavorings like cinnamon, nutmeg, vanilla, and maple extract.
- Create a side dish pilaf by combining vegetables cooked in a little olive oil with cooked grains and rice.
- Marinate cooked grains with salad dressings and sprinkle or toss into main course salads.
- Instead of using rice in a stir-fry, serve the meat and veggies on a mound of fluffy cooked quinoa.

Here are some basic tips to get started using grains in your browning program:

- Keep your grains in a cool, dry place away from heat and light, in a tightly closed container. I keep mine in glass jars in the cupboard. Properly stored, grains will keep for six months. If they smell musty or taste bitter, get rid of them.

- Use 1 cup of dry uncooked grain for 2 large or 4 small servings. Start with a ratio of 1 cup grain to 2 cups water.
- Start by measuring 1 cup grain to 2 cups water and then be bold. Rather than precisely measuring your grain and liquid, just cook your grains in a *lot* of water until they are soft and drain them in a colander. So even though we suggest specific ratios later in this section, be bold and experiment. If you are using the rice cooker, plan on 2–3 cups water for every cup of grain. Different people like different textures. More water makes them softer and a little mushier.
- Add salt after cooking your grains to avoid slimy mushiness.

How to Actually Cook Grains

Okay, so now you are ready to play. Buy grains at the natural foods store. You can either buy a small amount prepackaged or purchase larger quantities from the bulk foods section. Plan to buy about ½ cup dried grain for each person in your family and then an additional cup for planned-overs. Now you can take them home and cook them. Here are a few general cooking tips:

1. Rinse the grains thoroughly in cold water until the water turns clear. Strain them and examine them for dirt, small stones, or debris. Sometimes "brown" means dirt—you do not want your child to find a stone in her rice.

2. If you are cooking your grains on the stovetop,

either start the grain in cold water or bring the water to a boil, then add the grain and return the water to a boil. Cover the pot, reduce the heat, and simmer until the grains are soft. Do not lift the lid and look at the grains—letting the steam escape will prolong the cooking time. Don't poke them or stir them. Make sure there is enough water so you don't risk cooking it all away. This part of cooking grains requires some experimentation. If you are using your rice cooker, put the dry grains in with cold water, turn on, and leave the top on. Don't stir or poke even though you really, really want to.

3. Test the grains for doneness when the recommended time has gone by. I have a time with each different type of grain in the list below. Different grains have different characteristics—some, like quinoa, whole oats, and brown rice will be separate, while others, like amaranth, oat flakes, and millet, will be more porridge-like. Your family will tell you what they like. As you experiment, you will find that each type of grain has a number of subtypes. For example, different types of brown rice create very different flavors and textures.

4. Preroasting will enhance the flavor of almost any grain. Spread the grain you will be cooking in a skillet with ½ teaspoon olive oil. Heat over a medium heat until the grain is golden and begins to pop. Then add your boiling water and continue to cook.

5. Some grains do well with being fluffed after cooking. Remove them from the heat, and gently lift and separate them with a fork before serving.

Let me introduce you to some new grains. Don't be glazing over this section, now. You will be shocked to discover a whole new world. Be bold. And buy a couple of different kinds. Let your kids pick them and experiment. I am including grains that cook in a reasonable amount of time.

AMARANTH

Yield: 2½ cups cooked grain

> Use 1 cup grain to 2½ cups water.
> Simmer 20 minutes.

Amaranth is a gluten-free ancient Aztec grain. It has a sticky texture that is more like porridge when cooked. It congeals fast as it cools and can be lumpy if you don't eat it. Store uncooked grain in the refrigerator. Amaranth combines well with buckwheat, millet, and brown rice. It can also be popped like corn.

BUCKWHEAT (RAW)

Yield: 2 cups cooked grain

> Use 1 cup grain to 3 cups water.
> Simmer 15 minutes.

This is not actually wheat—it is a fruit seed and is gluten free. Since it has such a mild flavor, toasting it briefly in olive oil before simmering it in water perks up the flavor. It has a soft texture when cooked and combines well with quinoa, pasta salads, and winter squash.

BUCKWHEAT (ROASTED)

Yield: 2 cups cooked grain

> Use 1 cup grain to 2 cups water.
> Simmer 20 minutes.

Roasted buckwheat is also called kasha. It has a stronger flavor and a drier texture than raw buckwheat. It is great in pilaf mixed with rice, veggies, garlic, and other seasonings. Try coating 1 cup roasted buckwheat with 1 beaten egg in a heavy saucepan over medium heat. Cook, stirring, until dry. Add 2 cups boiling water. Cover, reduce heat, and simmer 20 minutes. Fluff.

KAMUT FLAKES

Yield: 2 cups cooked grain

Use 1 cup grain to 2 cups water.
Simmer 15 minutes.

Whole kernel kamut grain is pressed flat into a cereal like oatmeal. Add it to cookies or meat loaf. It is wonderful as a hot cereal, cooked with vanilla, chopped fruit, and nuts.

MILLET

Yield: 3 cups cooked grain

Use 1 cup grain to 3 cups water.
Simmer 15 minutes, then remove from heat and let stand, covered, for 20 minutes.

Millet is gluten free and is wonderful toasted in a little olive oil before adding water. It has a nutty flavor and goes well with curry dishes, soups, and salads. You can make breakfast porridge by adding extra water.

OATS

QUICK OATS

Use 1 cup grain to 3 cups water.
Bring to boil, stir, and simmer for 5 minutes. Serve as a cereal. Can get mushy.

ROLLED OATS

Use 1 cup grain to 3 cups water.
Simmer for 20 minutes. Use a soup thickener for pureed soups, in cookies, in hot cereal, or in shakes.

STEEL CUT OATS

Use 1 cup grain to 3 cups water.
Simmer for 30 minutes. Steel cut oats are made by steaming raw groats and cutting them with steel blades. The oatmeal has a very healthy and chewy, nutty flavor—it is great for morning cereal.

OAT GROATS

Use 1 cup grain to 3 cups water.
Simmer for 2 hours. If you presoak the groats overnight, you can reduce the cooking time to 80 minutes. Or you can slow-cook overnight in your crockpot and have a yummy whole grain breakfast.

QUINOA

Yield: 4 cups cooked grain

Use 1 cup grain to 2 cups water.
Simmer for 15 minutes.

This ancient Inca grain is loaded with nutrition. It has 50 percent more protein than wheat and more iron and calcium than most other grains. Rinse well before cooking, since the waxy coating on the grain can leave a bitter taste. Quinoa combines well with millet and buckwheat; it is great in soups and stews or as a side dish.

RICE

There are about seven thousand rice varieties worldwide, but they basically divide into white and brown and short, medium, and long grain. White rice is a basic "white thing." Short-grain rice is starchier than long grain and when cooked becomes stickier. It is good for puddings, cereals, and casseroles where creaminess is desired. Classic cooking uses short-grain rice in risotto, and in sushi and mochi. Long-grain rice separates when cooking and is dry, light and fluffy. There are a number of different long-grain rices. Basmati has a wonderful aroma like popcorn when cooked. Jasmine is classic for stir-fry. Texmati, grown in Texas, is a cross between basmati and a U.S. long grain. Wehani has red bran added and smells like buttered popcorn when cooked. Wehani is a nice choice for rice salads because of its wonderful color.

Some general tips for cooking rice:

Rinsing it before you cook releases the starch, and the rice will not thicken as it cools.

The general cooking ratio is 1 cup rice to 1½–2 cups liquid. Simmer for 45 minutes and let stand for 10 minutes before serving.

Toasting dry grains before adding the liquid adds nuttiness to the finished dish. Carrots, garlic, and celery add flavor.

You can pressure-cook rice, but it will not be separate, light, and fluffy.

WILD RICE

Yield: 2 cups of cooked grain

Use 1 cup grain to 3 cups liquid (I use chicken broth).
Simmer 45–60 minutes.

Wild rice is an extraordinary food. As I have learned about its role in the Native American tradition, I have been eating it more and more. Natural wild rice is unique from "paddy" or commercialized rice. It is a highly texturized, uneven grain that is medium brown in color and has a nutty smell to it. Commercial rice produces a long, consistent, black grain, which is harvested by machine.

We are carrying native grown wild rice in our store at www.radiantrecovery.com.

When I first started using whole grains, I tended to be cautious and serve them simply as a side dish like rice. Then I started to play and put them in all sorts of other things. A favorite breakfast is a cup of leftover grains mixed with 2 eggs and stir-fried. I think grains make browning fun.

8

Step Six:
Taking Out the Sugar

Now that you have the basics under your belt, your next task is to continue on this course and get completely steady before you move to the next step: taking out the sugar. You will master the changes you have made, continue to build the buy-in from your family, get skilled at dealing with the other folks in your life, and adjust some of the other factors that will enhance your children's healing. Let's take a look at these things first.

You have already made a *lot* of changes. Yes, they have been in baby steps, and yes, they have taken a while, but you are not in the same place you were when you started. This is not about doing a "diet." It is about making life change. This level of reorganizing your life needs some time to settle in. You want the patterns to become habitual and integrated. You want enough time not only for the impact of what you have done to settle, but also for the understanding of it.

After you are a few months into the program, pull out

your original journal—those "detective sheets"—and compare how things were to how they are now. Take a day or two to actually pay attention to how each child is eating. Think about your grocery and shopping habits and about the foods in your cabinet and refrigerator. Lots of change has taken place! After you have done this reflection on your own, call another family meeting. Share what you have noticed with the kids. Have them reflect with you and one another on the changes they see.

Take some time to congratulate your family on a job well done. These changes are *huge*. You all deserve major praise. And the more you congratulate your children, the more you reinforce that this is a positive lifestyle change, that it is a process and not just about getting off of sugar. If you honor the efforts your family has made and point out the benefits of these changes, you will help your children be more and more invested in the whole process. Children love learning new things. They are hardwired for it. You are not just dealing with food here. You are modeling ways of learning, ways of making profound changes in life patterns. As you teach them baby steps about making changes (in this instance, changing their eating), you are providing a skill set to draw from in everything they do. The key is simple: break your goals down into small enough steps so you don't get spooked, and do a little at a time.

What Do You Say to Others?

As you spend time practicing being steady, you are probably dealing with grandparents, spouses, partners, ex-husbands, friends, teachers, the teller at the bank who offers the lollipop, the school, the sugar industry. What do you say to

other adults who question the process? Originally, I had
thought about giving you a whole set of practice options,
including scripts to use. But I found in working with the
parents in our community that you don't need a script. As
you do the program yourself, you get clear. It is an organic
process. In the beginning, you don't have answers, you
can't make the arguments, because you don't know and
have not experienced "why" this process makes sense. But
as your body heals and things shift, you will have the
words just fine. Focus on your program and your kids' programs. And when you are settled and ready, move to Step
Six, and take out the sugar.

When you get to this step, you may find you have a
hard time with it. Your resistance may run deep. On an in-
tellectual level, it makes perfect sense. You believe in it,
you think you understand it, but something strange happens. You do it some, you cut back, but you can't really
follow through with a sugar-free household. Some of you
may worry about causing a rebound effect in your children.

> *I have two kids, a boy aged eleven and a girl who's eight.
> I worry about them feeling deprived and then making
> private vows to eat every piece of candy they can find.
> That's what I did. And I've been paying for it ever since.
> I want to apply the* PNP *[Potatoes Not Prozac] ideas to
> them and their diet, but it's taking a long time because
> they are so (dare I say it?) spoiled from satisfying their
> tastebuds with sweeter food.*
>
> *Lisa*

Your husband may fret that taking the kids off of sugar
will create kids like the ones who live down the street in
the "granola house"—the ones who are weird and not like

the other kids. And in fact there is a large body of literature that speaks to the issue of "deprivation." It says if you
withhold foods from your children, you just make them
seek them. You may have experienced that in your own
childhood. You may have had a mother who put you on a
diet, took you to a doctor for diet pills at age eleven, and
restricted your food. You know it did nothing except make
you more determined to get the foods you were not sup-
posed to have. And you certainly don't want to repeat that
story with your own children. Let's look at these fears and
myths.

If you just take their candy away and do nothing else,
they will feel deprived. Who wouldn't? Addicts are very
protective of the source of their supply. But you aren't
doing that. This is why we have been talking about the
buy-in for all these pages. You are going through a whole
long process of helping them register what sugar creates
and explaining why letting go of it makes them feel so
much better. They will feel empowered, not deprived. And
an empowered child has the capacity to be different. Yes,
she will be different from her friends. Yes, he may stand
alone. But you will be talking to them about being role
models, not freaks. You do this when you talk to them
about not smoking, not doing drugs. You encourage leadership and a willingness and desire to be different. Being
off sugar is no different and in fact may be even more
powerful. And they won't be "granola heads" because granola is too high in sugar anyway! They will be *your* kids,
and you will be mighty proud of what they are doing and
how they are being.

Step six can feel really, really hard. I have watched the
senior people in my community talk and talk and talk but

not be able to follow through with it. These were parents who were fully committed to the program. They believe in it, they are doing it themselves in a committed way. They are totally sugar free, but yet they simply could not move there with their kids. They got to the kid part and they waffled.

Getting Stuck

This truly baffled me. How could intelligent, informed, committed parents get so stuck? I started holding live chats every Monday night via our website with parents from all over the world. We talked strategies and recipes. We talked about schools and politics and ex-spouses. We talked about cutting down and making substitutions. Strangely enough, we never really got down to the topic of becoming a sugar-free household. Then one night we had a small group, and I decided it would be fun to just ask them: "So why is it you are so ambivalent?" We got to a key moment. One of the dads responded, "But what do you say to a four-year-old who is begging for ice cream and Oreos?"

Maybe it is because I am a grandmother with fifteen years in sugar recovery, but I would say, "I love you lots! We don't do Oreos and ice cream. How about a banana?" I truly understand how this is so hard for you. The message that sugar is love is profoundly embedded in every molecule of your body. The emotional attachment you have is shaped by every birthday, every trip to Dairy Queen, every holiday pie, every trip with dad for a Coke. You have been encoded with this belief. Sugar is love, sugar is comfort, sugar makes your woes go away. Sugar is a loving friend. Sugar is love.

My daughter has developed a sort of love affair with candy and sweets. For example, once in the car she was just musing about sugar and said things like "Mommy, I like things that are sweet" (with a lot of feeling). And she plays with blocks and pretends they are candy—carries them around in different containers. Once she carried around a book that had pictures of candy on one of the pages.

Audrey

The emotional love affair starts by age three. The biochemical response you have always had from being sugar sensitive is reinforced by advertising and the loving "pushers" who offer sweets everywhere. You have a sugar sensitive body; chances are you grew up in a sugar sensitive household. And chances are even higher that no family member was aware of any of this, so there were lots of sweets around. Your molecules love sugar. You were attached to it; it made you feel the world was okay, that you were strong and safe.

Because of this, you are sending two very contradictory messages to your own children. You want your child to love you. Giving sugar feels loving. You think, "I want you to have a 'real' birthday. I want you to know how much I care about you." So the first message is: I am offering you a sugar treat because I am offering you love, and I want you to value me.

The second message—which contradicts the first— comes in the face of sugar-driven behavior. Your child acts out, and you feel out of control. The whining starts, you are tired. The meltdown happens at church, and you want to crawl under the pew. It happens in the car or on a shopping trip, or an hour before dinner. Huge feelings surface. The rage that says, "I need you to stop this. I need you to stop whining. I need you to stop bugging me. I need you to stop embarrassing me. I need you to behave. I cannot stand this behavior!" In those moments, you don't care if sugar is bad for your child, you just hand it over in exchange for them to behave, you offer some ice cream. The second message is, "I am offering you a sugar bribe because you are bothering me."

Every parent I have talked with struggles with this problem. It is very normal. But if you can start to connect with the idea that the thing you are using to comfort and correct is actually creating the problem, you will find this step easier to take. If you remove sugar from the equation, you won't have those out-of-control moments with your child. Moving to sugar-free will have benefits that so outweigh your reluctance to say no and stand your ground that you will wonder why you didn't do it before.

Sugar As Love

If you begin to explore how you can make a core shift about sugar as love, you will be able to sweep an old belief from your molecules and bring in a new one. **Sugar is *not* love. Sugar is poison. Time is love.** Time spent with your children is love. Now you may be wondering what in heaven's name I am talking about. Go back and think about the memories of your own childhood. Do you think about birthday cake, or about the time Daddy taught you how to fill your bicycle tires with air. Or the time you went with Mom to work and wrote letters on her desk? Or when Mom read *Watership Down* in a big green chair with you sitting on her lap? Or tobogganing in the snow and falling into a snowdrift and having Mom's friend come and pull you out? When you made valentines or cooked breakfast for Mom and burned the toast? The day Daddy's friend played a board game with you on the floor for what seemed like hours and you laughed and laughed. When you walked the dog with Mom and your brother? When you went to the library and got a ton of books? Or the week you went to the northern lake with Daddy and fished in the early hours when the mist was still on the water?

These kinds of experiences are the very things your children most crave from you. If you are not medicating a sugar withdrawal tantrum or dealing with a whining child, you will *want* to spend time with your child. Your child will be the nice child you adore. Time with him or her will be the best of what parenting can be. As you really mull this over, the idea of moving to sugar-free is going to sound more and more exciting. You will get to the motivation part. You are ready. But the implementation of it may feel out of reach. The key is *not* to think about the idea of never having sugar in the house again. Just do one small choice at a time. Fruit one night instead of cake. Going for a walk instead of going for doughnuts when you are upset.

The anguish of following through on the sugar-free step lies more in the anticipation than in the actual doing of it. You may spend weeks or months or even years fretting about it. When you are clear, though, the actual implementation is quite easy. There are just a few key elements:

- You decide this is important enough that you want to do it.

- You are ready for your own sugar-free life.
- You identify the ways sugar gets into your house.

You are at step six now. Remember back to when you started, and look at your notes from that time. How much sugar did you find with that first review? How are things now? I suspect you have already made a lot of change. What is left now are the sugar places you are most attached to emotionally. When you are ready, you can take the last of the sugars out.

But remember, taking the last of the sugars out does not mean you just force it straight away. Think about the pattern you have built. You set the boundary, and then the children make choices within it:

- "Yes, we are having breakfast with protein. What would you like?"
- "No, we are not doing soda. What kind of water will work for you?"
- "Your lunch has to include protein. What shall we get?"

By now, you have had lots of practice with the commitment to making change. Taking out the sugars is simply an extension of the same way of making change that you and your children are now so skilled with. Call another of your famous family meetings and announce that you want to move to a sugar-free household. They won't be surprised and in fact have been waiting for this to come. Ask them to help you figure out what that will mean. Show them the Sugar List:

SUGAR LIST

barley malt	glucose	molasses
beet sugar	**granulated sugar**	polydextrose
brown rice syrup	**high-fructose corn**	**powdered sugar**
brown sugar	**syrup**	raisin juice
cane juice	honey	raisin syrup
confectioners' sugar	invert sugar	raw sugar
corn sweetener	lactose	sorbitol
corn syrup	maltodextrin	SUCANAT
date sugar	malted barley	**sucrose**
dextrin	maltitol	sugar cane
dextrose	maltose	turbinado sugar
fructooliosaccharides	mannitol	**white sugar**
fructose	maple sugar	xylitol
fruit juice concentrate	microcrystalline	
galactose	cellulose	

Overt Sugars First

Do not expect that you will take out every sugar in your household. Work on what we call the *overt* sugars first. I have made them bold in the Sugar List. The overt sugars are the ones we traditionally think of when we think of sugar. The *covert* sugars are the sneaky ones that get slipped in with funny names like fructooliosaccharides. But if you all learn what the sugars are, and have the label-reading expertise you now do, you can have a lot of fun discovering how artful food manufacturers are. When you read labels for the grams of sugar, don't be fooled. Legally, the only thing that needs to be labeled "sugar" is a very simple carbohydrate with two or fewer molecules. If the carbohydrate has three or more molecules in its sugar chain, it can be called a carbohydrate, not a sugar. However, your body and your children's bodies will respond to it as a sugar. The taste of sweetness evokes beta-endorphin. Whether it has two or three molecules in its sugar chain does not matter to your brain. So check for the carbohydrate count. If the list of ingredients includes any of the items on the Sugar List, assume that the carbohydrate count will give you a more accurate picture of the sugars in the food than the sugar count will.

Many health-conscious parents think sugars like molasses and organic brown sugar are better for their children than white table sugar. If your child is a sugar addict, whether a sugar has a little more nutritive value (as does molasses, which is high in iron) is really not important. Sugar is sugar. Sugar, brown or white, evokes the drug effect we are trying to curb. You may have wondered if it is better to pay a premium price for those special natural-foods graham crackers boxed with animals from the forest that are organic, low-fat, and produced with love. Nope, not from a sugar sensitive point of view. If you compare the labels, you will see that the sugar content is similar. This is intentional, just as the sugar content of a 12-ounce can of soda is almost always at least 38–40 grams. Consumers "expect" a certain sugar level, and whether it is provided by organic cold-pressed cane juice or old-fashioned white stuff doesn't really matter. What matters is the intensity of the "hit," not its source. If you find cookies and treats with significantly lower sugars, these are great alternatives. But read the labels, and don't be fooled by the artful hiding of the coverts. And remember that "natural" sugar is still sugar.

As you get ready to take out the sugars, have your children write down all their remaining sources of sugar such as:

Candy at Halloween
Cookies that Grandma brings
Candy bars at the movies
Sweets at a friend's house after school
Going out for ice cream
Yogurt pops

You have told them you want to move to a sugar-free household, and now you can ask them the best way to approach this change. Probably they will say they don't want to. Just laugh and say, "Of course not!" and keep on with the questions. Would it be easier for you simply not to buy the things that contain sugar? What about letting go of one sugar supply at a time? Would they prefer doing it all at once? Now, a couple of things may happen. The kids may get excited and come up with a pretty neat plan for taking the sugars out, one that you did not think of. (A number of our kids have done this. They essentially have left their parents in the dust shaking their heads while they rock into sugar-free lives.) Or they may resist this step and not participate. If that is the case, hold your ground, maintain a sense of humor, and do baby steps.

When we came home from our vacation to Pennsylvania, we went to the store to buy things for dinner. I told my four-year-old boys they could pick out a fruit to have for dessert. So, little addicts that they are, they ran over to the counter where they have all the "poison" and kept asking me "Hey, Mommy, is this okay?" I kept laughing and saying "Fruit. See the fruit over there?" Finally after a few times, I actually physically turned Pesach around so he was facing the rows and rows of fruit and said, "Fruit, pick a fruit." We came home with melon, purple and green grapes, and a pineapple.

After dinner I was reading this nature/animal magazine we get geared for three-to-seven-year olds. We were reading about raccoons and what they like to eat, i.e. fish. And the magazine asks a question, "So what do you like to eat?" Pesach pipes up and says, "Fish and poison!!!"

Naomi

Step six, in reality, is often a nonevent within the immediate family, but trouble arises with relatives and holidays. I will talk about that in just a bit. Remember that the steadier your children are at home with you, the more manageable those events and people will be.

Does having a sugar-free household mean that your children *never* have sugar? Nope. It means that your lifestyle is not centered on sugar. It means that over time you have less and less. It becomes less important. It is not the center of holidays or celebrations. You will lessen the focus bit by bit, and it will take more than one holiday season.

Two weeks ago I wrote about my experiment to put my house under NO MORE SUGAR. I had put a two-week time limit on it and wasn't sure what would happen after the two weeks. Those two weeks have me sold on keeping sugar out of the house, no doubt about it. My six-year-old has benefited so incredibly that it would be cruel to go back. She has slept better and had more control of her feelings and has just been a real joy, more than before! And the kids I (I also have a three-year-old) don't bug me for treats! Dinner doesn't revolve around dessert anymore—"How much do I have to eat to get dessert, Mom?" That's all gone.

But here is the kicker—they don't miss it! I partly knew this would happen because it happened to me when I went off sugar, but well, they're kids. After the two weeks we had a family meeting, and when I asked my six-year-old how she felt about it, she said she just didn't feel as good eating sugar and hasn't missed it. So there! Voilà! We are a sugar-free house!

Heather

Gradually, you and your children shift from *working* toward a "sugar-free house" to actually *having* it. Don't forget that each time you take something out, you are likely to have some crabby or moody behavior. It is, after all, drug withdrawal. And if your kids are crabby from withdrawal, give them a banana. Bananas are high in natural sugar and can take the edge off of withdrawal symptoms. You don't want them to suffer, and a little fruit will help bridge in the short term. Why a banana? It is quick, it is easy (and especially portable), and it seems to be just the right amount of sugar for the job.

Step six in *Little Sugar Addicts* is different from what many of you have read in my other books. The adult Step six is about detoxing when you plan and then pick a day to go off of sugars. You go through a physical process that takes five days; the first four days are very uncomfortable, but the fifth day is wonderful. But as I have been saying all along, your children function differently than adults. If you cut the sugars down gradually over time, the actual detox transition can be quite minor.

Some parents have taken this caution to mean they should *never* move to sugar-free, that it involves too much shock for the child. Nope, not at all. Generally it is too much shock to the parent in having to give up their role as a "feeder." This is a term that a very astute ten-year-old coined to describe her daddy's role in coping with his feelings. Daddy would be upset and take her out to have something sweet. She totally got the story. He did not. Lee's daughter got this as well:

> *The girls, especially my older daughter, has recently said, "Why do you want to feed us sugar all the time, Papa?" Wahoo, a small triumph! Keep on keeping on, and there are answers here that one could never find in a bottle of wine or a box of chocolates.*

One mom, Geri, talks about the "outside" feeders.

> *I stopped by the bank yesterday and the bank teller offered my son a red sucker. Didn't ask if I minded, just assumed it was okay, I guess. Fortunately, my son said, "I can't have this . . . too much sugar?" and I said it was. He put it down without a fuss—thank goodness. This was the first time he has been offered candy at the bank without my being asked if it was okay.*
> *On the way home, we also stopped at one of his friends' houses to play for a few minutes, and during that time, his friend gave him chocolate candy without my*

knowledge, which he ate. A few minutes later, he was out of control, screaming, crying, kicking . . . the whole nine yards. This continued until we got home and I got some real food in him.

This is big stuff. Huge! We are not just talking about making some changes to help your child have a healthy diet. This is about saying no to feelings about sugar that are deeply embedded at a core level and reinforced by billions of dollars of advertising. We are talking about your willingness to stand in the face of an overwhelming cultural belief, that sugar is love, that sugar equals goodness, and all the voices around you who tell you so. When your well-meaning mother says, "What do you mean, I can't bring her a birthday cake!" you will be ready with the right response: "No cake, Mom, but he would *love* to go to the zoo with you!" You have the skills to do this. You will help people like your mother see for herself, and then she will buy in as well. She will notice how happy and relaxed the kids are, and you will help her see the connection between sugar-free and this positive new behavior. And she will be noticing how relaxed and funny you are. (Or she may not, but your own program will help you deal with it just fine!)

9

Managing Holidays and Other Special Occasions

Though this program will become a natural, settled part of your family's day-to-day life, you may find that transitioning to sugar-free holidays is not easy, especially in the beginning. A great deal of how you can do holidays depends on where you yourself are in the process. For example, you might try having our Pumpkin Pecan Pie (see page 250) in year one and find the taste disappointing, but try it again in the second year and find it yummy.

Holiday food planning and preparation get easier over time, but they can still raise very old, very ingrained feelings about the role of sweet things in providing a message of love. And it will be little things, those rituals, their associations that get to you. For me, it took many years for the longing for green-iced Christmas cookies to fade. So you can take comfort by taking time. Don't feel bad if your ability to make these changes takes longer than you expect. They will creep up on you, and in year three you will be amazed at your progress.

Before we look at specific holidays and practical suggestions for each, let me share some general tips that our community parents found helped in the transition. After they had worked through their own feelings, the hardest part was the persuasive expectations of family and friends and schools and churches. These first suggestions simply offer a little buffer to give you some wiggle room. You can do them without people jumping all over you about why you are depriving your children or being weird. It helps to just show up with your own food.

- Suggest doing **potluck** at traditional holiday meals. If you aren't hosting, you can bring program-friendly food for yourself and your family. If you are just starting in the program and your family has yet to join you, your children may jump at the opportunity to have some "real" food and totally ignore what you bring. Make sure to bring what *you* will really enjoy. It is like a safety net that keeps you from falling if you arrive and find that all that there is to eat is white and sweet. I remember arriving at a baby shower without having planned for my own food. The food was laid out buffet style on tables that lined the walls. The "protein section" included some chicken and meatballs and took up about two feet; the desserts took up twenty. The rest of the space contained five different kinds of white pasta salad and what seemed like a hundred different kinds of Jell-O with marshmallows. No one really ate the chicken or meatballs, so I had plenty, but I was pretty light on my browns that day.

  This was a typical potluck menu, heavy on desserts and dishes like candied yams. The disproportionate

overload of sweets at such gatherings will seem daunting, particularly in the early stages of trying to get
your kids off sugar. It will seem as if sugar and white
things are everywhere and you cannot control what
to eat. But take heart because this will change over
time. You will become more and more confident in
your own problem-solving skills.

• **Ask for support.** You may assume that your parents
and siblings will not like the changes you are making,
and your sense that they think you are nuts may be
right on the money. But rather than being angry and
defensive about it and showing up at family gatherings and not being able to eat or going off your program, you can try a new tactic. Tell your family in
advance about the changes you have been making in
your house. Be kind and factual. Give them specific
suggestions about what will help most—like not offering Timmy soda and having sparkling water available. Ask if you can contribute some food that will
work for you and that the others will like as well,
such as Cheddar Cheese Mashed Potatoes (see page
237) or Apple Pear Crisp (see page 240). Bring great
food, and they will be forgiving about your plan. It
will be easier if you do not comment about what they
are eating. You know what to expect. You have been
eating in this family for your entire life. Let go of
your judgment and be nice. If you have what you
need for yourself and your children, wherever you
are in the program, you'll be better able to do so.

It is important to remember that as you go further into the program, it will initially be harder to be
in situations that are built around sugar. When your
program is new and still a little fragile, your tolerance

for partying with sweets will be low, and it will make you tense. You may feel like a newly sober alcoholic going to a party where drinks are the focus. As you become able to take care of your own needs, it will get easier. To some of you, the family dynamics of sugar addiction and alcoholism will be more uncomfortable the healthier you get. One parent told us the story of her sisters coming to visit. They asked for Coke, and she offered them sparkling water. They asked for rum, and she explained they were no longer drinking and had none to offer. They waited for sweets, and she offered them cheese and fruit. They didn't stay very long. She laughed and blessed them.

- **Bring your own drinks.** This little tip sounds sort of silly all by itself. But when everyone is partying, you don't want to have to walk around with ugly tap water in your glass. That would be pretty boring. It would make you resentful and cranky. If you bring sexy sparkling water that others may well envy, you will not only have your needs met, but you will have fun. And your kids will start seeing what it is like to make healthy choices with a great attitude.

Last year I held a conference here in New Mexico; when we planned the refreshments with the hotel, I told them we did not need soda. I knew who was coming, and 99 percent of the people were not drinking soda. Of course the hotel (like your family) simply did not believe this could be true, so they provided about 50 percent soda and 50 percent water. The first morning the water was gone and the soda remained untouched. The wait staff were shaking their heads. They simply had never seen anything like it. They all wanted to know who we were.

- When a family gathering comes up, you can suggest **eating out**. If you do a little homework, you can choose a restaurant that has program-friendly food. When our community parents get together locally, they do this. Recently a group planned for lunch in New York City. They went online and used the phone to look at menus and find out what was served. They called the restaurant and talked about choices. They picked a place that was not only program friendly but actually supportive of their food needs. This same group planned a breakfast for me the last time I was in the city. I arrived at the restaurant a little early and was startled to see that it was a place renowned for its desserts. The window was stocked with a hundred different kinds of chocolate things. But when it came time to order, the staff knew what our needs were and made wonderful suggestions; the chef made some special dishes just for the group. At the end of the meal the wait staff were intrigued to know what in heaven's name this group was. What could have been a stressor became a delightful morning.

This type of planning requires some real detective work. When I was staying in Maine for a month writing last year, I invited a group of my leadership team to come for a party. I planned a typical New England dinner for all of us. The local lobster pound served chowder that I had tried and found very tasty. I asked them if they catered and could provide that chowder in large amounts. No problem. The morning everyone arrived, I picked up the chowder, took it back to my little rental house, and made up the rest of the meal, including whole wheat buns and salad. We *loved* the chowder. In fact, we all had two and sometimes three bowls of it.

When I was clearing the table, I went into the kitchen and moved the container that the chowder had come in. I noticed a label on the side of the box. It seemed that the lobster pound had not made this chowder from scratch, as I had thought, but relied on a chowder maker to send it to them in bulk. Yes, so there I was reading the label in the kitchen: milk, *dextrose,* and so on. I thought I would simply crawl out the back door in embarrassment. I didn't. I went back in and told everyone that I had discovered why we all sucked down that chowder. And we laughed for the rest of the weekend as we noticed that every sweet thing in the world started calling our names. Humor goes a long way in the art of sugar redemption.

Let's look now at some specific holidays. The key issue for all of them will be to deemphasize the food and focus on the fun. Remember, abundance not deprivation. Add things in before you take them out. Take baby steps. The same principles you have been using all along will serve you well here.

Birthday Parties

Start by focusing on the point of the birthday party you are giving. You are honoring that your child was born and has grown. Spend time beforehand talking with the birthday child about why this is a special day. You know your children really well. See if you can think about what things and experiences other than sweet food might really be fun. Perhaps he is having a love affair with dinosaurs. Plan a trip to a local museum of natural history, and get a book or video about dinosaurs. Your five-year-old loves dancing. Take her to a local ballet, get her a little tutu and a CD of *The Nutcracker*. Your ten-year-old loves the out-of-doors. Make a special box and take her on a treasure hunt to the beach. Your twelve-year-old adores golden retrievers. Have a dog birthday party and invite all his buddies to come with their dogs. Be creative. Meet your child where he or she is.

If you haven't yet detoxed, go ahead and have the things you have always had, but plan to serve the sweet things *after* the real food. Protein first. Don't even think of having just cake and ice cream at three P.M. Even if you and your children are still on step one, don't set yourself up for failure. Now that you have some consciousness about sugar behavior, you won't be satisfied with a "straight up" cake-and-ice-cream party, I promise. Serve hard-core, dense protein first. Then have the cake and ice cream. Serve punch instead of soda, and water it down some. Offer juice and sparkling water coolers over ice. Make the games so much fun that the kids get caught up in the excitement of the activities and not the food.

Contrary to what many parents think, little children do not need cake to celebrate being one or two years old. We had an instance of one mother planning a sugar-free party for her son's first birthday. Her husband had a fit. He said, "I can't deprive my boy of a *real* party!" She decided not to take on that belief the week before the party. But she did compromise and say the "*real* party" food would be *after* she served a real lunch.

If your children are off overt sugars, or what I also call "big" sugars, you can make a sugar-free cake with them. Try the recipe out before the actual birthday so you are not faced with a disaster. I remember a specific incident where we planned an alternative sugar-free cake for my own birthday. It'd been many years since I have had a rich chocolate cake with white frosting on my birthday, so we were aiming for chewy, moist, and flavorful, and we decided to adapt a Martha Stewart recipe. My friend, who doesn't actually cook very much, came to my house for the big cake-making day. She unpacked the ingredients she had purchased and lined them up on the counter with great ceremony. She prepared the batter and the cake. What came out of the oven looked a little strange, like something that had died or been in the refrigerator too long. My son said it resembled a cow patty. I wondered how we would manage to eat it.

Everyone else at my birthday party slathered ice cream over their portions of the cake. I used applesauce. The cake was pretty strange—actually it was awful, but it was so funny and my friend's effort had been so valiant, that, I didn't really care that I didn't have "real" cake.

Don't let anyone tell you, "You won't miss it after a while." Of course you will. It's like losing a dear friend. But over time things shift. Your attachment will move from the drug (the cake) to the love (the people). The joy will be in the party, the celebration, family, and friends. The taste of cake won't be the standard of love. But be sure to try out any recipe you plan to adapt *before* the big day!

Another alternative is to simply not serve cake. Here is Laurie's experience:

For my birthday, my friends made me a delicious fruit salad, with lots and lots of perfect fresh fruit. They had "extras" to put with it, like whole grain crackers, yogurt, and cheeses. I truly did not miss the cake at all—nor did anyone else! There was not a crumb left after the party . . . unlike the half-cakes we had to try to palm off on someone at the end of the day. I have always remembered this, because I actually preferred the fruit salad to a birthday cake (and believe me, it takes a lot to make me choose fruit over cake)—it was so delicious and refreshing. Most of all, it showed how much my friends cared about me and took my food plan seriously. Friends like that are priceless.

Laurie touches on the heart of the change you will want to make. Move from food to people. Your children love to play—capitalize on that. You will have to deal with parties in your house and then parties with your children's friends. Jennifer was concerned about what to do:

We're going to a birthday party on Sunday afternoon at McDonald's, from one to two-thirty. I've been giving some thought to the recent posts on this topic, and about how I should talk to my girls about it and get their input about the sweets that will be there. The problem is, I don't have a clue how to do this.

Should the goal be to get them to not have any cake and ice cream? Or have a few bites and stop? Or share a serving? Okay, I realize as I am writing this that these are my ideas not theirs, which is defeating the purpose of getting their input. I could really use some pointers here.

I suggested to Jennifer that the key is to talk with her children and do problem solving ahead of time. The key is to help them make choices, not to control their food. Take baby steps. Listen to how Gail managed an ice-cream social.

> We had the annual ice-cream social last night at the elementary school. It's a fund-raiser and works like this.
>
> One ticket for each family member. The ticket entitles you to one piece of pizza, one soda, one baked good, and one ice-cream sandwich. Not too program friendly!
>
> Here's what we did. We bought four tickets, to support the school. We gave each girl two tickets and asked them how they'd like to handle things. We started talking about it on Thursday so it wouldn't be a surprise!
>
> Together they decided to bring water bottles (i.e., skip the soda), each have two pieces of pizza, throw away the ice-cream coupons, and take a baked good home for dessert for the next day (today). Would I like them to skip the baked good also? Sure. However, I allowed them to make the decision, and I think all things considered they made a good one.
>
> So one cupcake and two cookies came home. Lindsey had a friend sleep over, and they decided to have a snack, cheese and a cookie and some milk! I let it be. In a way, I thought it was better for Lindsey to have one cookie last night rather than two today—at least now they are gone.
>
> Kayla put her cupcake on a napkin on the kitchen table. I decided I was not going to enable her, so I didn't wrap the cupcake. This morning it is on the napkin on the table, as stale as can be. I'm sure it will be headed for the trash can.
>
> Eddie and I volunteered during the social. First we poured soda. There was no water unless you brought it.

Many children asked for water so I poured it for them from my bottle and then went into the school and re-filled it. Funny, their parents were of the attitude, "Oh, just take a soda." I was clear to give any child who asked for water, water. I will let the PTA know that they need to add some options!

Then we served pizza. Again, here some parents only bought one ticket, so their kids were entitled to only one slice of pizza. I was eyeballing the children and putting two on their plates, or giving any child that asked for it an extra slice. Figure there's not much protein in a slice of pizza, an extra slice would be good for most.

I think the whole key at our house was letting the girls talk this one through.

School parties, sleepovers, and functions will meet you at every turn. These are where the rubber will hit the road in your child's program. Gail has given you some great ideas for transforming the school fund-raiser, so let's think about when your child is asked to go to a friend's house for a sleepover. Lots of sweets and chips and soda will be served. He may feel uncomfortable about being different. What to do? Think about what Gail suggested. Talk with him beforehand about how to handle this so he can think through alternatives. Perhaps he would like to bring sparkling flavored waters and chips and dip. Here are some other suggestions from Connie, whose daughter was faced with many invitations to sleepovers, birthday parties, and other social events involving foods.

My daughter was very social and went to many parties. In my experience [the kids] didn't really care what the food was, just so there was a lot of it and they could "eat with abandon" the whole time. Here are some ideas that worked for us.

If the families are new to each other, I might call the other mom and ask if my kid could bring snacks, too. Then if the parent sounded savvy, I might add that we like to stay away from super whites and sugars.

If the kids are old friends, just send fun bean dip, salsa, and cheese along with the kids. Fancy "Talking Rain" flavored waters. Turkey Jerky. Then if your kid wants to choose healthy food that night (and I bet he won't always), then at least it's there.

If your kids are a little older than eighth grade, buy fresh berries and serve with fresh cream from a CO_2 canister from a fancy food store. Boy, is that fun.

Breakfast the day after the sleepover can really be a nightmare. With that one, we found it was really best for [my daughter] to have cheese or cottage cheese to augment the white-o-rama that was sure to be offered. Otherwise, an icky breakfast after such an exciting night could make her feel awful by evening.

What Connie did was think through the variables. At first blush it seems that if your child wants to be part of the crowd, there are few choices. But the one who brings the food is well thought of, so have it be your child and send really good food. One time Connie sent a pot of really yummy sloppy Joe mix and very fresh whole grain buns. The kids loved it. Call the hosting mom. Perhaps she can add egg burritos (or just eggs) to the morning menu. It never hurts to ask. Offer to stop by with a load of tortillas and scrambled eggs for all the kids in the morning. More work for you? Of course, but planting seeds is always a good thing.

Halloween

Many of the parents originally felt stumped by Halloween, the queen of all sugar holidays. But they are getting creative. Vicki is making changes in the treats she offers:

> *Last year I bought little things, like pencils, cheap Harry Potter glasses, the Halloween long scary fake fingernails, things from the birthday gift aisle at Wal-Mart, etc., and put them in little gift bags tied with a ribbon. My son helped me put them together. We just did a few each night for about a week. I spent a little more than I would have on candy, but I didn't feel guilty about handing them out. I gave a bag to a few friends' kids, and they loved them, so I am assuming that the kids at the door like them, too.*

Here are some other goodies our moms give out:

- small packets of pencils
- microwave popcorn
- small toys from Oriental Trading Company (you can buy these online or through their catalog)
- small bags of pretzels
- small bags of Goldfish
- packets of cheese or peanut butter crackers

Gail actually "buys" her girls' candy—she purchases the candy from them in exchange for cash and they use the money to buy things they really want, like music CDs. She got a number of the other parents intrigued by this idea. Vicki liked it a lot:

> For the past two years, I have bought back my kids' candy. I will give them fifteen dollars each, and they would much rather have the money than the candy. Originally, I let them pick out five pieces that they could have with meals, but not all at once. This year I am going to tell them that I will buy all their candy for twenty dollars. Even the five pieces are making me uncomfortable now. Of course that doesn't mean they won't sneak some while they are out trick-or-treating, but at least I'm making a dent!

Melanie now does a sugar-free Halloween party with finger foods and games. She holds a costume contest, and then the kids all make jack-o'-lanterns together. No one even thinks about the candy anymore. Maggi does the same in a big way:

> I decided that we would make our Halloween tradition about the pumpkin carving and the costume. That way there is a special trip to pick out the pumpkin, carve it, and eat dinner in the dark by pumpkin candlelight on Halloween.
>
> The other thing I had always wanted to do was to teach my son how to sew—he picks out his costume, we go to the fabric store, pick out patterns, he chooses the fabric, and we sew it together (that means I do 90 percent of the work, and he sews a few straight seams, pins the pattern, and pins fabric . . .).

This has worked great, as he has costumes for dramatic play that are really nice that he uses all the time throughout the year. The costumes this way are a little pricey and very labor intensive for Mom, but his cool midnight blue with silver trim wizard costume will be treasured for many years.

Janie raised yet another alternative. She and her family simply changed the rules for Halloween.

We decided we are going to go to the Grand Canyon! We will stay a couple of days and then drive the whole way back on Halloween. So we will miss the stupid holiday altogether and not have to worry about it. I will, of course, talk to them about all the fun we will be having on our trip, and all the fun things we will be doing instead of trick-or-treating.

Christmas

It is a big shift to plan a sugar-free Christmas. It is very, very hard the first time around, but it gets easier with each one you do. When you are early in your program, you might want to try just one little baby step that fits where you are. If you try our Pumpkin Pecan Pie (see page 250) before you have gone off of sugar, you will find it pretty bad. But try making the Cranberry Chutney (see page 219) and see what you think. Eat the sweet stuff after your meal rather than at midday. Plan one low-sugar dessert for yourself. Leave fretting about the foodstuffs for another year. Just do what you do and start the process of shifting the emphasis from food. Spend an afternoon with your children making ornaments rather than cookies. You will still have cookies because Mom or a neighbor will bring them, but you can start a new tradition. Remember, before you take things out, you add them in. Changing holidays is the same as doing the program—baby steps and abundance, not deprivation.

For years I missed those Christmas tree sugar cookies with the green frosting. But I don't miss them anymore. Now I have New Mexico Christmas Eve with thousands and thousands of little luminarias, those paper sacks filled with sand and a lighted candle at every house. No Christmas cookie can match the feeling of a perfectly still southwestern night with those special candles lighting the way. No cookies can replace the joy I feel as I look through fifteen years' worth of special ornaments for my tree. When I take out the box, I unwrap each one and remember that the Santa in a yellow slicker came from Maine and the ball with the dolphin came from Maui. I don't miss the cookies anymore. Or the pie or the Droste chocolate apple in the toe of my stocking. And in fact, without the shrine of food, I value the holiday more.

There are some holiday recipes in the back of the book that will give you a sense of meal alternatives. Christmas can be sugar free and a lot of fun. As with other major events and holidays, don't expect an instant or total shift to sugar-free. It will take time. Each year all of you in the family will be willing to do more change. The change will be incremental, and your new traditions will replace the old sugar-laden ones, and after a couple of years, you will have made incredible progress.

Thanksgiving

Thanksgiving is a funny holiday. We associate it with all that dessert stuff after dinner. The dinner is really quite program friendly, unless Auntie Maud is still making sweet potatoes with brown sugar and marshmallows. But oh, the desserts, the desserts.

But think about the real Thanksgivings that you have now. Sometimes everyone has too much to drink, or sometimes siblings fight, or sometimes the pressure of being back at your mother's is unbearable. Much of the stress of Thanksgiving is about a group of sugar addicts or alcoholics being cranky, sloppy, or teary. We often create a romanticized myth of the day, and the reality is not so fine as the fantasy. But as you get steady and relaxed, things start to change. You will get clearer and enjoy visiting with relatives, or in some instances you'll see how unhealthy the environment truly is, and you'll realize you do not need to spend a lot of time with them. Your program will help you be clear.

I stopped having expectations about how Thanksgiving should be and started to enjoy the heart of what it meant. A couple of years ago I suggested to my adult children that perhaps we might all get together and go someplace fun for Thanksgiving as a family. As they live on the East Coast, I called my ex-husband who lives in Boston to ask about ideas for where I might set up this outrageous idea. He said, "Well, if you go someplace within driving distance of the kids, you can use the money you would spend on airfare for the place to stay." He is a logical kind of guy. We talked some more. He said, "Hey, why don't Patty [his wife] and I come along, and we can share the expenses."

All of us ended up going to Nantucket for five days. We rented out a bed and breakfast. We biked and sang and shopped and ate, all in different configurations. The day we biked out to the ocean, the younger ones took the long route, and those of us who are over fifty went at our own pace. But we met by the sea and watched the sun dropping low over the sand. We came back and sat by the fire. My middle son brought out his guitar, and we sang and talked and laughed. Yes, we ate a fine meal on Thanksgiving Day, but did we care about dessert? Not one whit. We started a new tradition. And it had nothing to do with the food we used to have, nothing. Instead, we went to the core of what Thanksgiving means to all of us—family—and we have built on that.

Now, if you have small children and are just getting started with the program, it is going to take some time to ease into this approach. Listen to how Heather is making small steps:

Well, my family left today, and my kids are a great big mess. Oh boy. I made some advances, but not as many as I'd have liked. One of the last things my mother-in-law said (and mind you, this was after a week of conversations on the matter) was "Oh, here's some crackers [white saltines], they don't have sugar, only salt. They are white, but oh well." Sigh.

But the good news is . . . we are back to a sugar-free household. I threw away all the goodies, and after a few days of aftermath we will be back to the fun, kind kids I have grown used to.

What I did like about all this was knowing why my kids were acting like they were. My six-year-old was in

tears and saying awful, horrible things to her sister, but
we talked about why she was feeling that way.

Easter

Easter was always my favorite holiday. I now know it
was because I gave up sugar for Lent, and then Easter
morning truly felt like a resurrection. Forty days of fasting
from sweets, and then a whole basket of jelly beans and
stuff was about as close to heaven as you can imagine.
Did I care about anything except the clothes and the
candy? Nope. But the program changed this. Without the
candy, I started exploring what Easter meant to me as an
adult. Easter vigil, the candle, the music, the sunrise over
a purple New Mexico mountain. And eggs are very program friendly! Mary, one of our moms, loves eggs, too.

> *Last Easter we had an absolute blast coloring real eggs! I*
> *got this huge pallet of jumbo eggs, and we boiled and*
> *colored them all the night before, which took hours. The*
> *next morning we had an egg hunt in our backyard, all*
> *real eggs, none filled with candy. The whole thing wasn't*
> *focused on sugar, and it was great. My kids each got 1*
> *small chocolate bunny, and they couldn't touch it until*
> *after a real breakfast. I also found these plastic eggs*
> *filled with toy cars and got them each one. So it was al-*
> *most sugar free, and it was great.*

I still love Easter baskets. Every year I make them for my
children, and I spend a whole day making old-fashioned
Easter eggs. Last year I did this with my four-year-old granddaughter, Madison. I got special coloring at the store, and

we set out to make really cool eggs. Though they didn't quite come out as we planned (the color didn't work and oozed all over the table), we still had lots of fun. And a funny thing happened: when Madison went back to Daddy's that night, she instructed him how to make eggs. They stayed up late coloring eggs and hiding them, and her interest in Easter candy and chocolate treats shifted to something new. We make Easter baskets with no candy, no chocolate rabbits. Rabbits, yes, lots of rabbits, but no chocolate. I spend a lot of time thinking about what wonderful things to put in the basket I send off to my daughter. A box of tea, a package of seeds, some bubble bath, a new pen, a compass, a whistle, a favorite book, tiny rabbits. No sugar, but *lots* of love. And I get the time of planning and finding and creating and packing and mailing. Way more fun than going to Wal-Mart for the candy. And the baskets she makes for her own kids are changing, too. They have less candy and more fun little things.

Rosh Hashanah

Naomi has shared the same ambivalence and struggle. Traditionally Rosh Hashanah is a celebration of sweetness, and honey is a huge part of it. An apple in honey is the usual tradition.

> I'm not sure how I'm going to handle the honey situation with regard to my kids who have been off overt sugars and most coverts for two months (well, besides what their *rebbes* give them). It is a tradition that is so ingrained that I honestly feel a bit ambivalent about it. My family accepts that I don't eat the honey, but I think it is

more because I am diabetic than because of my doing the program. I was thinking that a no-sugar-added all-fruit spread might be a nice alternative to honey. I know that since I am ambivalent, my husband will never agree to it. I have a few weeks to work on this, though.

I was thinking that it is nice to reflect on the sweetness that life has when one is doing the steps. I was thinking how absolutely sweet my life has become, how the radiance is much sweeter and more special than honey.

Naomi is making baby steps, and like most of our parents, she is shifting her awareness to the meaning of the holiday rather than the literal food traditions.

Purim

This Jewish holiday is filled with sugar-laden food. The kids dress up in costumes, and the adults give food gifts to one another. Last year Naomi made some sugar-free whole grain treats and gave those away. She made an apple cake with whole wheat flour and applesauce as the sweetener, and she made whole wheat hamantaschen, a traditional pastry, with apple butter as the filling. This year she is thinking she might use fruit-only preserves for the filling. In dealing with the goodies for the kids, she is planning to use some of the same tactics that our other parents use for Halloween and give small toys or trinkets instead of food.

As you read through all of these approaches to holidays and special events, you can see what happens when you begin to think of taking the sugar out; the true meaning of the celebration comes into focus. It doesn't have to be a perfect step or a finished one. Just becoming aware creates a positive change in the right direction. No matter what your tradition or what the holiday, the principles are the same. You take baby steps and make small changes to start with. You expect the shift to be gradual and take time, not to be absolute or instantaneous. You emphasize your relationships with family members and close friends, and you adopt a loving and playful approach to the holiday with your child. You put the emphasis on the time you spend together and not on the foods you eat. This gets easier and easier as *you* are doing the program yourself. It is no longer a source of stress, and you will find new ways to express your love. Once you step into this way of relating to special times, you will get hooked. So will your children. Your creativity will flourish, and you and your kids will have a blast in the process. The sugar and white things of holidays will become a thing of the past.

10

Refining the Program
for Special Needs

Kids who are further into the sugar sensitive continuum than others have some special needs. These are kids who have been diagnosed with (or are at risk for) problems such as diabetes, obesity, attention deficit disorder (ADD), and oppositional defiance disorder (ODD). Here is an overview of how these conditions are related to sugar sensitivity. You will see that a major component of these diagnoses are simply further iterations of sugar sensitivity and that doing the food can have a profound and positive impact on children who struggle with these imbalances.

Addressing these special needs is really no different from what you are already doing. You will simply work with your child to take the core program a little further, emphasizing some specific changes over others. You do not have to be scared by any of these conditions, though until you understand how biochemistry creates them, they can seem overwhelming and baffling. The behaviors associated with some of these imbalances seem to come out of nowhere. Perhaps it is as if you are living with a little time bomb, a miniature Dr. Jekyll and Mr. Hyde. The whole family walks on eggshells lest Annemarie has a bad day or Mike gets locked into one of his fits.

You no longer have to be ashamed or embarrassed about having an "off the wall" child or an overweight child. Adopting an attitude of resolve and dispassion is one more piece of taking care of business. In this chapter I will walk you through what is going on with your special needs child and what you can do to resolve the problems. I firmly believe that under every sugar sensitive child with an extra "problem" is a sugar sensitive child who is smarter and more creative than average. You are going to get a bigger pay-off for the extra work you and your child will be doing.

Diabetes

There are two types of diabetes, type 1 and type 2. Historically type 2 was considered "adult onset," but in recent years many children have been developing it. Both types involve a problem with high sugar levels in the blood. In a healthy body, the sugar is carried to the cells and is taken out of the blood by a hormone called insulin. Insulin acts like a little key in the cell door. It opens the door, and the sugar goes in to be burned for fuel. In type 1 diabetes, it is as if the key got lost. The pancreas just doesn't produce the insulin your child's body needs. In type 2 diabetes, it is as if the lock is rusty and the key doesn't turn the lock very well.

Treatment for a child with type 1 diabetes requires taking insulin. But getting the timing and amounts right is very tricky because it requires balancing what and when the child is eating, how much and how she is exercising, and her emotional state. Managing type 1 diabetes is hard and takes practice. Doing the program helps the rest of the child's body stay in balance, and that makes sorting out the insulin needs a lot easier.

I am going to focus primarily on type 2 diabetes because its development is so tied to diet in untreated sugar sensitive children. Type 2 diabetes occurs when your child's body becomes resistant to the insulin it produces. When your child has lots of sweet things and lots of white things, his little body has to produce more and more insulin to try to cope with it. Over time the hormone system just sort of gets tired and says "forget it" and stops responding to the insulin. This type of diabetes is very responsive to changes in the diet. Doing the steps of the food program will make a huge difference for your child. One of the biggest culprits contributing to insulin resistance is a diet high in high-fructose corn syrup. And guess what is used in soda! So just taking the soda out is going to have a huge impact on your child's vulnerability to diabetes. As your child eats fewer sweet things, her body releases less insulin. Less insulin means the cells become more responsive to it.

So the plain old vanilla steps are just what your diabetic or prediabetic child needs. You simply have to be more rigorous with a diabetic child than with a regular sugar sensitive child. But as you look to control the insulin that is spiking in your child, there is one key thing to pay attention to: diabetic children can get depressed easily. Many people once thought this was simply a function of getting the diagnosis. They didn't realize that it is a very direct consequence of the biochemical changes in the body. Healthy brain functioning requires some insulin to get the tryptophan from the blood up to the brain to the serotonin factory. When you are trying to control insulin levels to reduce insulin resistance, you may not know about the serotonin piece. So you want to be vigilant about sweets and white things, but you also want to find a carbohydrate snack to give your child that does not spike blood sugar but moves the tryptophan to the brain to raise serotonin levels. We use a baked potato in the *Potatoes Not Prozac* program for adults, but the potato effect may be too intense for children, who have naturally higher levels of serotonin. A rice cake may be the ideal option. Your child's blood sugar levels will guide you in finding the ideal solution for the serotonin adaptation.

Here are a few other factors to think about with your diabetic child. There seems to be a very high correlation between diabetes and celiac disease. Full-blown celiac disease means that the body cannot digest gluten—which is found in many grains, especially wheat. The gut says "whoa, no way" and spits it out. So the nourishment from whole grain wheat that you think is a really healthy food doesn't get absorbed. If the body isn't getting the food it needs, the blood sugar can drop, making the natural volatility of a sugar sensitive child even worse.

It is likely that your child does not have full-blown celiac disease, but he may be sensitive to wheat. This adds another variable that you haven't thought of. If your child is diabetic, think about cutting down the amount of wheat foods your child is eating. Use rice cakes instead of wheat crackers. Get wheat-free bread. Check www. livingwithout.com as a great resource. This may be daunting at first because wheat, like sugar, is everywhere. Don't even think of starting to take wheat out until you are firm in your own program and your child is very settled with the steps. But after extensive research, I am convinced it is a factor, and probably a big one, for the diabetic child. So, put it in the back of your mind as you and he refine his program. As you start reading labels, maintain your sense of humor and do what you can.

Exercise and Childhood Diabetes

The other major component of diabetes treatment is exercise. For the child dealing with diabetes, exercise can mean life or death. In an experiment done in Israel, a group of scientists tested the effect of exercise combined with different kinds of diets: one was high-calorie with no exercise, one was high-calorie with exercise. The scientists reported: "None of the animals in the high energy/ exercise group became diabetic, whereas all of the animals in the high energy/no exercise group became diabetic." Read it again, and note those words *none* and *all*. Exercise matters.

Exercise may be tricky because often diabetes goes hand in hand with obesity, and an overweight child may resist exercise for both physical and emotional reasons. Let's take a look at the obesity part and see if we can weave these together.

Obesity

Having an overweight child is a complex and emotionally charged task for any parent. You may feel a lot of shame and anger about it, but you don't want to upset your child and add to what she is already feeling, so you try to keep your mouth shut. Or you have lots to say about it and you nag him constantly. Or your husband has lots to say about it, and you try to balance his negativity so you act as if it is not important. Or you may be overweight and feel it is not fair to bring it up with your child because you can't deal with your own weight. Or you may have been fat as a child and have huge feelings about it that you do not want to bring down on your child. Or you may have residual pain about it and do nothing but push your child precisely because you want to spare her the pain you had. As I said, it's complex.

Your own doing the program will have a huge impact in your being able to sort out how to approach your child's weight. You will get "clean" and be able to separate your feelings, judgments, and history from the functional issue of what to do and how to do it. I want to support you in the process by giving you a road map. If you follow these instructions, I guarantee you your child will lose weight, and you will change the course of that child's life in ways you cannot now imagine.

No Dieting!

First off, you are *not* going to put your child on a diet. Don't even think that. But you are going to talk about what is going on. Your child knows she is "fat." No matter what you have done to try to convince her that it is not important, that she's pretty and lovable and all that, it doesn't matter. She knows she's "fat," and all that stuff you have done to try to ease the pain of it simply makes her feel that *you* are in denial and she has to hide her feelings from you. So start talking. Do not be afraid to use the word fat. It will actually comfort your child because she knows what she looks like, and that is the word she uses to describe herself. Using the word *fat* rather than *over-weight,* or *heavy,* or *plus* helps to take the charge off it. If you have feelings about being fat, share them. Sugar sensitive children are extremely intuitive. She already feels what you feel, and if you are saying something contrary to what you really feel, she knows. And the dissonance sends the message that being fat cannot be spoken of. If you were fat as a child, tell her. Talk about what is real. When you get clothes and have to go to the plus sizes for children, acknowledge it. Tell her you know this is really, really hard. And talk about how easy it is when you are feeling bad to turn to food for comfort. Talk about doing the food as a solution. You know this story. You can be her biggest support.

As you are doing the food plan and the steps, do not talk about it being a diet to lose weight. Talk about healing the body. If she starts getting excited about losing weight, deemphasize that part for now. Stress healing and balance. Tell her the weight-loss part will come, but that first you want to heal the reason she got fat. And then you progress through the steps just the way you do with any of your children. Doing this food plan creates balance and healing, and weight loss will follow.

Let's talk a little about the biochemistry of your child's weight. Sugar sensitivity means that your child can gain weight disproportionately to the number of calories she eats. A sugar sensitive child can eat the same number of calories as her normal friend and she will gain more weight. This fact is extensively written about in the obesity literature but is not widely known in the popular literature or addressed by most doctors. So your child may not be hugely overeating. Do *not* assume she is sneaking food or lying about what she is eating.

I learned about the dramatic differences in bodies when I was writing a book on weight loss called *Your Last Diet!* I discovered that the same strain of mice, known in the research world as the C57 mouse, who loves sugar and alcohol also gains weight. C57s tend to become insulin resistant. They get fatter because the sugar in the blood can't be burned and gets stored as fat. The sugar-loving C57 mice are hardwired to gain weight in their abdomen, so they get tubby tummies. Even when they exercise, they gain weight. It was shocking to me to find that differences in biochemistry affect gaining weight. The weight gain was not a function of eating too much. Science has not formally established that human "strain" differences correspond to mouse strain differences relative to sugar sensitivity, but it has clearly shown that some people are predisposed to obesity and diabetes. I have no doubt that sugar sensitive people are the human equivalent of the C57 mouse strain, and I expect this will be shown in the scientific laboratory within five years.

All this scientific information can be a huge comfort to you in dealing with your child. I will repeat the message I have been giving you throughout the book: you are not a bad parent because your child is overweight. You simply did not know about the effect of her biochemistry on her weight gain. Like a C57 mouse, your child has hardwiring that triggers weight gain, depending on how and what she eats and how she exercises. By making changes now, you can prevent a lifelong struggle with her weight and self-esteem.

Heal the Sugar Sensitivity First

There are a few key issues for you and your child to know to create weight loss. Heal the sugar sensitivity by doing the food program. As you and your child get that part steady, tweak it a little by paying attention to fats. Take out fried foods. That is all you have to do. No counting, no fretting. Don't even think of a low-fat diet—that is not what you want. Growing brains *need* fat—they especially need the "good" kind of essential fatty acids that are called omega-3 fatty acids. Cold-water fishes such as tuna and salmon are rich in omega-3s. You can either serve more fish, or you can give your child some fish oil, one of the best fats there is for overweight children. Pediatric fish oil comes in little capsules or in liquid form, available at most natural foods stores. I went on a hunt to find good oil for the kids in our community, one free of heavy metals and that did not taste fishy. If you cannot find something you like locally, check our website store (www.radiantrecovery.com) for several kinds of children's oil.

Some of you may have kids who are not yet obese but are getting a little pudgy around the edges. With these children, you simply work to cut down the snacks that are higher in fat (such as cheese and peanut butter) and use protein sources that are leaner, like broiled chicken rather than chicken nuggets and reduced-fat cottage cheese or milk. And get them exercising. I will talk about this more a little later on.

Some of you may have really obese kids. As you work with these children to create a plan for change, remember that the most important issue for them is *you*. Let me explain what I mean. Recently a highly publicized court case in New Mexico involved a three-year-old child who was extremely obese. The child had been put on a low-calorie liquid diet but had not lost significant weight. As a result, the state removed her from her parents, calling the girl's morbid obesity a case of child abuse and neglect. There was a huge outcry in support of parental rights, met by an equally loud call for the child's "protection." I listened to the interviews with the parents and saw them as sincere, concerned individuals who honestly had no clue what to do for their daughter.

After much legal wrangling and negotiation, the state finally agreed to return the child to her parents. Amid a crowd of reporters' cameras and microphones, this darling, very overweight three-year-old came home to her mama and daddy. I will never forget the image of that smiling child walking with her daddy; one of his big hands was gripping hers while the other carried an eighteen-pack of Coke. I don't think anyone saw the incongruity of that, but I still see it. This is addiction. The state can take your child away and you do not make a connection to your own life or what you are eating. This is a child who will be given gastric bypass surgery at age eleven. And to my mind, pediatric gastric bypass surgery is the biggest example of medical failure in the world. It is the most unacceptable solution to childhood obesity I can imagine. The people who offer that solution have no other answer. But you do.

Those of you who are here reading this book are fearlessly looking at these issues. You are seeing that they are all intertwined. A fat kid is not a kid in isolation. A fat kid is a kid whose biochemistry predisposes her to gain weight. Her sugar sensitivity is not controlled, and her addiction progresses. The impact of her food choices creates insulin resistance. Insulin resistance means sugar doesn't get burned and gets stored as fat. The fatter she becomes, the more insulin resistant she is. It is a vicious cycle. And it sets her up for a lifetime of anguish, yo-yo dieting, and serious health problems. Your intervention now will change all that. Not only will your child lose weight, but she will be spared the profound imprinting of being "less than" that comes with being a fat kid. So *your* healing is at the heart of your child's healing.

Get Them Moving

Let's look at the biggie for children who are overweight—exercise. Most overweight kids watch a lot of TV or play computer games for many hours or sit and read by themselves. Most normal-weight kids ride their bikes or play sports more than children who are overweight. Do you know what your child does after school? Most parents do not. Perhaps you have not made a connection between their weight issues and how they spend their free time. You are dealing with your own busy life and haven't really considered this. If you are sugar sensitive, this is one more thing that will shift for you as you do your own food program. People who are lost in sugar addiction tend to be self-absorbed. I surely was. I was all caught up in my own drama, my own issues, and I assumed I had well-adjusted kids. I didn't really spend a whole lot of time thinking about what their days were like after school.

If you have an overweight child, it is safe to assume that he or she spends more time sitting than moving. Many parents who know this just tell their kids they need to exercise. But telling such a child to "go exercise" is like telling a sugar addict to "just say no." It doesn't work. "Big" kids don't exercise, because it is uncomfortable or shameful for them to do so. They get out of breath easily, they do not feel connected to their body, they feel ashamed of having less clothing on in group situations, and they get picked last for the teams. They feel klutzy and are often uncoordinated. Exercise generally does not represent something fun or something they aspire to do. The solution to your child's exercise plan is very much like the solution to the eating plan. You start by creating a buy-in and you do baby steps. And you don't simply tell them to do it, you do it with them.

Many families in our community have started walking together. At first it seemed like a small thing, an after-dinner walk for maybe twenty minutes to half an hour. Everyone loved it, in part because the heavy kids could keep up. It was not a big deal, and it got them moving. And once you get moving, the body remembers that it likes moving. So then our families started biking together. They started taking weekend trips and vacations that involved physical activity rather than passive sitting.

If your family is superbusy, you may wonder where "moving time" will come from. The answer is simple: take it from the sitting time. This means that TV and computer time give way to walking, biking, playing catch, or just playing. As I said before, doing the exercise is like doing the food. You can't just tell the children to do it, you need to do it, too. Healing your children means committing to sharing their journey in a different way.

What About Television?

Perhaps you have seen articles and heard about studies that connect obesity to watching television. This may be another source of uneasiness for you as a parent. You may wonder if you created the problem. You like having your kids quiet and entertained. You park them in front of the TV as a way to have some quiet time. You are exhausted and have no downtime, and the TV provides a respite even though you know it has a downside. Here is the exciting part. As you do the program, you are not going to feel so overwhelmed. Instead of turning on the TV or simply spacing out while the kids turn on the TV, you are going to be able to say, "Hey, how about going outside and riding your bike?" You may even surprise yourself and say, "Hey, let's all go for a bike ride!" Baby steps. Or instead of providing fast-food snacks while the kids are watching TV, you will offer water and carrots, whole grain crackers, and cheese sticks.

Shifting the amount of TV your children watch is very much like what you have been doing with the food. Sit down with the kids, and have them do a log of what they watch in a week. Count up the hours; take a look at the content. You might want to get a copy of the book *"Mommy, I'm Scared"* by Joanne Cantor, a really good resource for making sense of how your children respond to what they see on TV. You may be surprised to learn how deeply some of the images affect your children. Not only does violence affect them emotionally, it affects them physically.

Just as you have done with the food program, get the facts and work from there. Negotiate a reasonable number of TV and computer hours for the week, and have them work out a transition plan. You do not want your children to simply shift from TV time to computer time. As you take the poll, count "screen" time regardless of what kind of screen it is. Count Web surfing time, Game-Boy time, computer game time. Talk with your kids about what is healthy interactive time and what is time lost. Talk with them about the content of what they watch. If they are overweight, watching action adventure or violent material will contribute to their being fat. Yep, it's true. Content that is high arousal makes the body release a stress hormone called cortisol. Cortisol helps to keep them fat. Weaning your children from TV and computer games is not easy, but you need to know how it fits into the fat equation.

There is also a huge emotional pay-off in getting an overweight kid moving. These children are ashamed of their bodies. They often do not have exercise clothes that fit. Sometimes denial sets in, and they don't want to tell you that what they have in the drawer is too tight and they are not comfortable wearing it. Or else the shame factor is so big, they are wearing clothes they swim in. So take your child shopping for some athletic clothes that fit and are in style. Remember when you had to wear those awful gym clothes? Resolve that you are going to give your child something a whole lot better. Make it a quest. Find cool stuff that fits. You may ask yourself why would this matter, what difference it will make. By going on this quest, you are saying it matters. You are confronting the shame factor without making it worse. You are reinforcing the idea that there are solutions—that you don't have to hide, that shame can be transformed. You are saying it is not a big deal to be heavy, it can be resolved, and you are willing to put your money where your mouth is. You are reinforcing the fun of making a change, making healing the focus, making moving easy and exciting. Getting good exercise clothes is like getting good food. It will have a profound and positive impact on your child.

Attention Deficit Disorder

Attention deficit disorder can affect the way your child processes information, and in those instances where it exists, medication can be life saving. However, I think it is impossible to make a diagnosis of ADD until you know the impact of your child's diet on his behavior. Many physicians and counselors will tell you that diet has no impact on the brain. Most often they will reference the role of sugar in ADD. They will say that countless studies that have shown that sugar is not a problem in ADD. I am going to challenge that. I have analyzed most of these studies, and I can honestly tell you that how a study is designed will have a huge impact on the results it gives. Sugar is like an opioid drug that quiets the brain in the short term. So if you give a child a big dose of sugar, then measure whether he is hyperactive, I guarantee you your study will show he is not—it will show he is quiet and attentive. But if you measure when he is in withdrawal or when he has skipped breakfast and then had a soda, you will get different results. Test a child who has Pop-Tarts for breakfast and soda and chips for lunch, and you will get a child who cannot focus or pay attention. Take a child who has had no protein in two days except some Chicken McNuggets, has downed a liter of diet soda, and is now sitting in front of the computer playing games, and you will have a diagnosis of ADD.

Sugar Addiction Is Real

One other interesting finding comes from the lab of Dr. Bart Hoebel, a professor at Princeton University. Dr. Hoebel is very interested in sugar addiction and was the first person to actually show that rats could get addicted to sugar. He also discovered that amphetamine-sensitized animals are hyperactive following a taste of sugar. He suggests that sugar may be acting on the same system as amphetamine to sensitize them to sugar. He noted that repeated doses of amphetamine can set up an appetite for sugar that lasts for at least a week. So the amphetamine-like drugs you are giving your sugar sensitive children diagnosed with ADD may be making their sugar cravings worse and contributing to the hyperactivity you are trying to treat. It is backward.

In our current culture doctors, educators, and parents rush to medication far too early in the game. Literally thousands of parents have reported to me that their child's symptoms of ADD simply vanished when the food changed. No drugs, no counseling, no major therapeutic intervention. This is not to say there are appropriate and very useful times when medication is a powerful tool. But with ADD I do not think you can know what times those are until your child is steady on a healing food plan. Do the food with an ADD child, and you will see what is underneath all that "stuff." Maybe you have a child who needs to move, who learns by doing, not by sitting. Maybe you have a child who is very, very bright and simply finds most of the stuff around him incredibly boring. Perhaps your child's learning style is incompatible with the teaching style of his fourth-grade teacher. Get a copy of Mel Levine's book *A Mind at a Time* and do a little homework on different ways of learning. Added to the food program, Levine's approach can make a very big difference for an ADD child.

Your children may already be on drugs. How can you know if drugs are the best solution? What options do you have? These are highly complex questions with no easy answers. But I do know one thing beyond a shadow of a doubt. If you and your child do the food and go through the steps, a major biochemical shift will happen. Doing the food will allow you to make a far more informed judgment about what is right for your child. Both of you will be able to sort it out from a place of stability and will know what is right for you.

Oppositional Defiance Disorder

You will recall the story of my two grandsons on the infamous drive to New York. If you have a child like these two, the ones who are gifted and funny but can become little monsters, and you don't know about the biochemistry, their behavior can be terrifying. It is almost as if these children enter an altered state, something you cannot reason them out of. All the "calming" tips from the experts do not work. The fits embarrass you. When it happens in church, you feel as if the entire congregation is watching and wondering what is the matter with you as a parent. Your ex-husband is sure that your parenting skills cause it, since he "controls" it and your child does not act out at his house. He, like some of your friends, tells you to "just discipline that behavior out of him," and that your beloved three-year-old has you "tied around his finger." Now, in your heart of hearts, you *know* the behavior is not just manipulation, but everything you have tried is not working, so you question everything you trusted about your skills as a parent.

As they get older, these children are diagnosed as having oppositional defiance disorder and are put on medication. This new category has been added to the *American*

Psychological Assessment Manual as a "pattern of negativistic, hostile, and defiant behavior lasting at least 6 months, during which four (or more) of the following are present:

1. often loses temper
2. often argues with adults
3. often actively defies or refuses to comply with adults' requests or rules
4. often deliberately annoys people
5. often blames others for his or her mistakes or misbehavior
6. is often touchy or easily annoyed by others
7. is often angry and resentful
8. is often spiteful or vindictive

Notice that I said this is a *new* category. I think there is a very clear reason for this behavioral dynamic: untreated sugar sensitivity at its worst. In the last ten years, the increase in consumption of junk foods and soda has climbed astronomically. But if you don't know that your child's behavior is biochemically based and you are told he has a serious psychological problem, you are going to be one overwhelmed parent. And your child will be boxed into a diagnostic behavioral category that will shape how he is treated for his entire school years. Your child will be branded as a bad child who is oppositional and defiant, stubborn and willful.

The good news is that you do not have to go there. You now have a set of tools that can reverse this biochemistry and totally alter the direction of your child's life. ODD children have a very, very small tolerance for blood sugar drops: they go from okay to empty in ten minutes, have no reserves, and go into an altered state. The Hulk emerges, and you all are in big trouble. A diet with sugar and white things makes this margin between a manageable child and a defiant child even narrower. And when the Hulk is stomping around, it is impossible to remember the Snapple for lunch or a breakfast without protein. Without knowing the biochemistry, you just focus on the behavior. And if your health-care practitioner or counselor does not have a sugar sensitive frame of reference, they will say that medication is the solution. They will say your child has no impulse control and needs to be on Prozac. Before you go there, treat the sugar sensitivity and *feed* this child.

ODD children need to eat every few hours. Enforcing a "no food between meals" rule is a recipe for a disaster with them. Breakfast, then snack, then lunch, then snack, and perhaps another snack if dinner is running late. Give them food before bedtime, and make it protein food. If they wake up in the middle of the night, they are not being manipulative, they do not have an incipient eating disorder, they need to eat. Make a shake with whey protein powder and chocolate almond milk, and leave it by the bed in a covered cup. Have them shake it and drink. Give them cheese sticks. Don't worry about them getting fat. Feed them.

I have worked with a number of sugar sensitive mothers who are overweight and concerned about their children having to suffer what they have. So they are very cautious about food portions with their children. They are not withholding and restrictive; they are sincerely trying to do the right thing. But they don't see that weight is not the issue with these kids. These kids are high burners. They are sucking up every ounce of food and using it.

When they say they are hungry, they *are*. Feed them. Move them along to step six sooner. Be really vigilant. Give your ex-husband a copy of this chapter. Send it to school to your child's teacher and principal. Send food, send enough, and include protein. And watch something happen. It will knock your socks off.

Now, if your child is already on medication, hold the meds steady, do the food and talk with your prescribing doctor. As the behavior changes, you may just find that you don't need the medication. *Do not just take your child off it*. Take the book and flag this section, share what you have observed, and working with your child's doctor, make a plan to taper your child off the meds. Join our parents' group online. Come and share the journey with the other parents who are doing this. Hear the success stories; hear the profound changes we have seen with these kids just by doing the food. Be comforted to know that this is not about some weird, unrealistic far-out program that you cannot possibly do; it is about cheese sticks at night and water for lunch.

Mike, Kevin, Grace, Tyler, Matthew, Emma, and Margaret—children of our community parents—are just like your children. Having been on this program, their lives are not the same, and your children's lives will not be the same either. The change won't happen in a week or a month, but three years from now you will feel the way Jennifer and I do. You will be thrilled that the solution was food, just food!

11

Life After Sugar

You have made some awesome progress in getting through these concepts and mastering the Six Steps. There is a Seventh step—the fun step, Life After Sugar. This step brings the enjoyment and effect of all your work into focus. I want to offer you a preview of what life can be like after doing this program. Here is Jennifer's story about her daughter Clara. It speaks to the heart of what "doing the food" can create for you and your children.

> When Clara was a baby, I knew about sugar sensitivity and wondered if she was or wasn't sugar sensitive. I knew I was, and I knew her older sister Emma was. I hoped that Clara had escaped the wrath of the sugar sensitive biochemistry. As she got older and her diet expanded and included more variety (including sugar), I looked for the signs that I thought I knew: hurt/sensitive feelings, cravings, withdrawals. I didn't see them . . . I thought her biochemistry was different! (At the time, I was trying,

failing, and trying again to move through the steps my-self. Sugar was still in our lives.)

Around the age of two and a half, she started waking up in the middle of the night. One of two things would happen. She would either be wide awake but calm, or she was badly tempered and couldn't be pleased (at all). Neither option was fun. If it was the first, I would put her back to bed over and over. Each time she would come back in my room, wide awake as could be. I would plead with her to "just go back to sleep!" Some nights she was awake for hours. If it was the latter, she was in-consolable . . . she wriggled, she cried, she thought she wanted one thing or another but never wanted anything at all. It was draining. She would eventually fall back to sleep, exhausted. So would I.

Eventually, she started articulating that she was hun-gry in the night. I really didn't believe her, quite hon-estly. (After all, she'd been sleeping for two years through the night without being hungry!) My sugar-fogged brain thought she was manipulating me, just trying to get an extra snack. (After all, that's what I would have done when I was a kid.) For a long while, I resisted giving her a midnight snack. Eventually, I gave in. My offer was always a cheese stick (for the pure beauty of no crumbs in bed)!

Pretty soon I discovered that on the nights that she woke up, a cheese stick got her back to sleep in no time. It took less than five minutes to lie down with her while she ate, and then she immediately went back to sleep. That meant that I could go back to sleep myself! Life was good!

But then there were mornings in which her dis-position was utterly horrendous. I remember holding my breath when she came down the stairs in the morning, waiting to see if she had a smile or a scowl on her face. The smile meant we would start the day on a good note. A scowl meant that we were in for a loooooooonnngggg, difficult morning. (If Clara wasn't happy, NOBODY was happy!)

Over time, it wasn't just the mornings in which Clara's disposition became abominable. There were explosive episodes throughout the day. She could transform from a contented playing child to a sour, defiant, stubborn, unreasonable monster. She defied us; she had to have things her way (or not at all); and she was oblivious to where she was, who she was with, or the activity of the moment. It was a state of being, and when she got this way, it felt impossible to get her back to "normal." It always took a long time.

Of course, she wasn't like this all the time, either. She was often funny, silly, sweet. And there was no doubt that she was smart. She was mechanical, always wanting to know how things worked, extraordinarily verbal, and always "seeing" things that seemed beyond her age.

It was like she had two personalities, and the dissonance between them made me extraordinarily uncomfortable. As a parent, I couldn't help asking myself, "What am I doing wrong?" I hadn't connected the dots; I didn't know it was food related. I thought it her personality, and I wondered, "If she's like this now, what will she be like when she's eighteen? Twenty-five? Fifty?" I fretted about her future. I didn't know what to do.

Feeling rather desperate, I started posting Clara's behavior on the Radiant Parents list. It was the best thing I could have done. Over time I gained a whole new understanding of what Clara needed. A clear picture emerged from the scattered dots. Keep her fed; *don't wait for "empty." Give her a bedtime snack with protein. If "empty" happens, fill her up first; handle the discipline later. Each tip that I learned and employed helped Clara's coping mechanisms and our family life.*

Clara is now four. She wakes up smiling every day. She loves to make people laugh by doing silly little dances, making funny faces, and saying funny things. Her creativity has blossomed through her stories, paintings, coloring, and new inventions. She can concentrate on an activity for hours. She hardly ever scowls.

The secret? I make sure she is fed regularly every day: three meals and three snacks, with protein at each one. Is life perfect? Of course not. Do I mess up? Yep. But now I know how to fix the mistakes. If Clara becomes frustrated, I know "empty" is near. If she wakes up in the night, I know a snack will put her back to sleep. If she decides not to finish her breakfast, I know that an early snack will be in order. When we go out, I always bring water and a snack. These adjustments are so simple, so manageable, so doable.

Our journey has been long, it has had its ups and downs, but it has been oh so worthwhile. I no longer fear my daughter's moods or fret over her future. I am thrilled that the solution was food, just food! It sounds unbelievable, but it is absolutely true.

Jennifer and Clara are people just like you and your children. As you gradually move into this new lifestyle, you will notice that some remarkable changes are happening. Connie calls it the "happy baby syndrome": "It's like getting the big-kid equivalent of the 'easy baby.' You know, the one that smiles, sleeps well, plays well, goes everywhere, and rarely fusses."

I think Connie is right on target. I see it all the time. Instead of squabbling all the time, your kids are actually playing with one another. You overhear delightful interactions that you could not have conceived of in your "old" household. It is as if your family connects now. Addiction does funny things and impairs the capacity for relationship. The emotional drive for connection goes into maintaining the addiction, not into maintaining the relationships. If you have a whole family of sugar addicts, they spend a lot of time coping with the biochemical effects of feeling really good while they are "using," and feeling really bad during withdrawal. And generally every addict in the family is on a different schedule. It is as if a whole bag of marbles gets loose and bounces every which way. It makes life chaotic. But when the entire family starts doing the food, something happens. Instead of having a group of individuals all zooming around, you get a coherent whole—you get a family and family members who start thinking about one another.

Addicts are very self-absorbed and have to work really hard to pay attention to the needs of others. As the mother of addicts, you had to work really hard to keep things together. But Mom herself was not there. Now, no one ever talks about this. You were under so much pressure to maintain the illusion of your family being okay that you could never talk about feeling so tired you could not see straight or feeling that there was no room to breathe.

You *love* your kids, and you felt completely overwhelmed and desperate for your own psychic space. Having children and running a household is a hugely demanding job, no matter what. For you, trying to do it in the throes of sugar addiction was so hard, it was scary. You felt as if you were just coping. And you couldn't tell anyone about it. Who was there to tell? If you spoke what you really felt, you were judged an inadequate parent. Why were your kids out of control? you wondered. Why did they throw fits in public and embarrass you beyond belief? When you didn't know the reason, in your heart of hearts you believed it was your fault.

You held all those feelings inside. You couldn't talk about them. Now that things are getting better, it is safe to revisit all that. It is important to do this because I want you to really see it was not a function of your inadequacy. It was a function of your biochemistry. You were a collection of biochemically unbalanced people all doing the best you could. Now something else is happening. The love that has always been there now has a chance to work its miracle in a different way. You all can connect and enjoy one another. Now you are getting a house of funny, goofy, creative, smart kids having fun with a mom who is present, relaxed, and loving.

This connection doesn't go away. Your journey into life without sugar is really way more than "without." It is about holding the biochemistry of your sugar sensitive family steady and then growing the spirits of everyone in it. When people first start the program, this idea is inconceivable. This is what feels like the Norman Rockwell myth. But now, after this commitment, after this change, you know exactly what I mean. And it keeps getting better. The other shoe does not drop. Even after a vacation when everyone wobbles and you start growling with one another, you remember what life is like doing the program. And you come home and you put back the pieces, and three weeks later you have grown from it and learned more skills and more tools for the next time.

You keep growing into this outrageous idea that there is no failure; there is no black and white, no right and wrong. There is simply supporting balance and from that place a healthy and informed understanding of how to live. People who start this program think it is about getting the sugar out. They have no idea of the pay-offs that come with it. Sometimes it may seem like a miracle, but it is not. Doing the food is not magic; it simply gets the static out of the way. Doing the food gives you the capacity to be a focused, loving parent.

Even the early struggles and frustrations with the feeders will simply go away. You get funny, you set boundaries. Your ambivalence melts. Being on board ripples out from your kids to your spouse and partner to your parents and friends. It is not forced or angry, it is clear and consistent. Your kids actually say no to things that make them crazy. They say, "Hey, Grandma, we don't eat that stuff." They take lunches to school and actually eat them. They carry water. They don't whine and beg for soda.

This isn't about obesity or diabetes or ADD or behaviors. This is about going to the heart of the issue and resolving it. And you have done that. You have done that by changing the food—an act so remarkably simple that all the experts in the world missed it—one parent in one family with one kid having breakfast on time, having enough food, having protein, and giving up sugar.

Now, that sounds sort of amazing, yes? But here's the scoop. When I started working with parents, I thought the kids would feel better and get more settled. I didn't understand the nature of healing a collective addiction. But listening to all the parents and hearing what was happening knocked my socks off. At first I thought, this level of change simply could not be. It had to be a function of a few really committed parents, a skewed sample of people who were so committed, so willing, and so diligent that it couldn't fail. But that wasn't the case. Everyone who did the program, who stuck with it and kept working at it, experienced the same miracle. Doing it imperfectly, doing baby steps, groping toward making it happen, everyone got the same results. It didn't matter how old the kids were, it didn't matter if Daddy or the other adult in the house was on board at the start. It didn't matter if Mom was working or was at home or if the family made a lot of money. It didn't matter if the kids went to public school or private school or were home schooled. It didn't matter if the kids were boys or girls. In the homes that did the food, the miracle happened and got better over time.

In the beginning of this book, I made a promise to you. I told you that if you did this program, things would get better. I promised you would get your child back. Now you know that promise can be fulfilled beyond your wildest dreams. I know that you and all the parents who are doing this can enjoy this time with your children. You can have what you dreamed of when you had your children. And that is really cool!

Recipes

Many times recipes are added to a book as "filler" and are not particularly useful to the reader. I once read a kids' book that had a recipe for Spinach Artichoke Pie and Eggplant Dressing. Those recipes didn't sound like something I would make for my grandchildren. All the recipes I have included here are for dishes I have both cooked and eaten. And all of them are kid tested. I wanted to give you ideas about real foods you can actually use with your family. My own staff calculated the nutritional information.

BASIC RECIPES

GEORGE'S JR. SHAKE

BASIC SHAKE

1 cup cold milk (cow, oat, almond, or rice)
George's Jr. Shake Mix (according to your child's size.
    Check the label)
Frozen fruit to taste

APPLE CRISP SHAKE

1 cup cold milk (cow, oat, almond, or rice)
½–1 sliced apple, skin on
George's Jr. Shake Mix (according to your child's size.
    Check the label)
2 teaspoons dry roasted almonds
½ teaspoon cinnamon

PUMPKIN/SQUASH/SWEET POTATO SHAKE

1 cup cold milk (cow, oat, almond, or rice)
¼ cup canned pumpkin
¼–⅓ cup George's Jr. Shake Mix (according to your
    child's size. Check the label)
1 teaspoon carob powder
1 teaspoon cinnamon

BERRY SHAKE

1 cup cold milk (cow, oat, almond, or rice)
¼ cup frozen blueberries or strawberries
George's Jr. Shake Mix (according to your child's size.
    Check the label)

BANANA SHAKE

1 cup cold milk (cow, oat, almond, or rice)
1 small frozen banana (freeze without the peel)
George's Jr. Shake Mix (according to your child's size.
    Check the label)

Put all ingredients in blender, and blend for 30 seconds.

KATHLEEN'S BAKING MIX

1½ cups mix

¾ cup oat flour
¾ cup brown rice flour
½ teaspoon salt
2 teaspoons baking powder (nonaluminum)
½ teaspoon baking soda

1. Combine all ingredients.
2. Use as directed in recipes calling for Baking Mix.
3. Leftover mix can be stored in refrigerator tightly sealed for 1 week.

Prep time 3 min.; cook time 0 min.; beginner skill
708 calories, 20 g protein, 137 g carb, 15 g fiber, 1 g sugar,
8 g fat (1 g saturated fat), 2264 mg sodium

KATHLEEN'S BAKING MIX WRAPS

6 servings (2 wraps each)

1 cup Kathleen's Baking Mix (see above)
1 cup milk
1 egg, lightly beaten

1. Heat griddle or skillet. Lightly coat with cooking spray.

2. Stir all ingredients into a medium-large bowl until well blended.

3. For each wrap, pour 2 tablespoons batter on hot skillet, spreading to make a 6-inch crepe. Cook until top is slightly dry. Turn and cook until bottom is golden.

4. Cool, then serve with your favorite filling.

Prep time 5 min.; cook time 15 min.; beginner skill
25 calories, 1 g protein, 4 g carb, .4 g fiber, 0.3 g sugar,
1 g fat (0.1 g saturated fat), 25 mg sodium

DROP BISCUITS

6 servings (each serving 2 biscuits)

1 ½ cups Kathleen's Baking Mix (page 213)
6 tablespoons chilled butter
1 cup milk or buttermilk

1. Preheat oven to 450°F.

2. Place Baking Mix in a medium-size bowl. With a pastry blender or 2 knives, cut the butter into the baking mix until the mixture resembles coarse cornmeal.

3. Make a well in the center of the mixture and add the milk all at once. Stir until combined, but do not overmix.

4. Drop batter from a large spoon onto an ungreased cookie sheet, spacing the biscuits about 2 inches apart.

5. Bake 10–12 minutes or until lightly brown.

Prep time 5 min.; cook time 15 min.; beginner skill
236 calories, 5 g protein, 25 g carb, 2 g fiber, 2 g sugar,
13 g fat (8 g saturated fat), 278 mg sodium

Note: Biscuit flavors can be easily changed with the additions of various ingredients. Experiment by adding any of the following:

SAVORY BISCUITS

1 ½ teaspoons dried herbs such as basil, oregano, thyme, sage, chives, or rosemary

⅓ cup crumbled or grated cheese such as cheddar, Parmesan, Roquefort, or Swiss

4 tablespoons sautéed onion and garlic mix

3 tablespoons diced ham, cooked bacon, or cooked sausage

SWEET BISCUITS

1 teaspoon cinnamon with ½ teaspoon vanilla extract

½ cup blueberries

½ cup chopped nuts with ¼ teaspoon almond extract

½ teaspoon maple flavoring

OVEN COATING

4 servings

2 cups crushed Triscuits or rye crackers

1 teaspoon granulated garlic powder

1 teaspoon onion powder

½ teaspoon paprika

½ teaspoon cracked black pepper

½ teaspoon salt

1 tablespoon parsley flakes

2 cups plain low-fat yogurt, whipped until creamy

1. Combine all ingredients except yogurt. Place mixture in Ziploc bag.

2. Dredge food you wish to coat into whipped yogurt, covering all sides.

3. Place food into plastic bag with coating, close bag and shake to coat food.

4. Oven-bake at 375°F until cooked through.

Prep time 5 min.; cook time 0 min.; beginner skill
413 calories, 13 g protein, 56 g carb, 7 g fiber, 9 g sugar,
15 g fat (3 g saturated fat), 730 mg sodium

Note: This coating works well for chicken, firm white fish, or shrimp.

QUICK PIE CRUST

Pie dough for 1 crust (6–8 servings)

> *¾ cup oat flour*
> *¾ cup brown rice flour*
> *¼ cup canola oil*
> *6 tablespoons cold water*

1. Combine flours together. Add oil and water. Mix lightly till soft dough forms.

2. Let dough rest 5 to 10 minutes before rolling out.

Prep time 5 min.; cook time 0 min.; beginner skill
197 calories, 3 g protein, 23 g carb, 2 g fiber, 0.1 g sugar,
10 g fat (1 g saturated fat), 2 mg sodium

CRISP POTATO CRUST

1 9-inch pie shell (6–8 servings)

> *2 cups grated potatoes, packed*
> *½ teaspoon salt*
> *1 egg, beaten*

¼ *cup grated onion*
olive oil

1. Preheat oven to 400°F.
2. Set the freshly grated potatoes in a colander over a bowl. Add salt, toss, and let sit for 10 minutes. Squeeze out excess water.
3. Place the potatoes in a bowl, and add the egg and onion. Toss to combine well.
4. Pat the mixture into a well-oiled 9-inch pie pan, building up the sides of the crust with lightly floured fingers.
5. Bake for 30 minutes. Brush the crust with a little olive oil to crisp and color it.
6. Return to oven for another 15 minutes.
7. The shell is now ready to be used as a crust in your favorite quiche or other savory pie recipe (such as chicken-mushroom pie, cauliflower-cheese pie, scallop pie).

Prep time 15 min.; cook time 45 min.; learning skill
55 calories, 2 g protein, 9 g carb, 1 g fiber, 2 g sugar,
2 g fat (0.4 g saturated fat), 204 mg sodium

SPINACH-OAT CRUST

1 9- or 10-inch crust (6–8 servings)

2 *tablespoons olive oil*
12 *ounces fresh spinach, finely minced, or a 16-ounce*
    package frozen spinach, defrosted and squeezed dry
½ *teaspoon salt*
½ *cup brown rice flour*
¼ *cup oat flour*
¾ *cup regular rolled oats, crushed*
¼ *cup grated Parmesan cheese*
dash nutmeg

1. Preheat oven to 375°F. Lightly coat a 9- or 10-inch pie pan with nonstick cooking spray.

2. Heat oil in large skillet. Add spinach and salt, and sauté quickly over medium-high heat until fresh spinach is limp or frozen defrosted spinach is dry and heated through.

3. Remove from heat; add remaining ingredients and mix well.

4. Pat mixture into prepared pie pan. Mold crust with your fingers.

5. Pre-bake 15 minutes.

6. Crust is ready to be filled as you desire.

Prep time 15 min.; cook time 15 min.; learning skill
173 calories, 7 g protein, 22 g carb, 4 g fiber, 1 g sugar,
7 g fat (2 g saturated fat), 318 mg sodium

COBBLER CRUST

Pie dough for 1 crust

   1 egg, lightly beaten
   3 tablespoons milk
   1 tablespoon butter
   ¼ teaspoon vanilla (for dessert cobbler only)
   ¼ cup oat flour
   ¼ cup brown rice flour
   ½ teaspoon baking powder
   Pinch salt

1. Combine egg, milk, and butter together in a medium-size bowl. If you are making a dessert cobbler, add vanilla.

2. In another bowl, combine flours, baking powder, and salt. Add dry ingredients to wet, and mix just enough

to combine so that all ingredients are moistened. Do not overmix.

3. Use crust as directed in whatever recipe you work with.

Prep time 5 min.; cook time 0 min.; beginner skill
434 calories, 15 g protein, 48 g carb, 5 g fiber, 3 g sugar,
20 g fat (10 g saturated fat), 612 mg sodium

CRANBERRY CHUTNEY

10 servings

> *4 Valencia oranges, peeled and cut*
> *rind of one orange*
> *4 cups apple juice*
> *2 pounds fresh cranberries*
> *1 ½ cups walnuts*
> *1 teaspoon cinnamon*
> *pinch nutmeg*

1. Cut up the oranges and put them in a saucepan. Add the rind of one orange. Add apple juice and simmer for 15 minutes.

2. Add cranberries and walnuts.

3. Simmer for an additional 15 minutes until mixture thickens.

4. Add cinnamon and nutmeg.

Prep time 10 min.; cook time 30 min.; beginner skill
232 calories, 6 g protein, 32 g carb, 6 g fiber, 23 g sugar,
11 g fat (1 g saturated fat), 4 mg sodium

BREAKFAST FAVORITES
(Good for Lunch and Dinner, Too!)

BREAKFAST ROLL-UP

1 serving

>   1 6-inch whole wheat flatbread, pita, or tortilla
>   3 eggs
>   ¼ cup shredded mozzarella cheese
>   1 tablespoon toasted onion flakes
>   salt and pepper
>   ½ cup meat, fish, or chicken
>   ½ cup veggies, potatoes, grains, beans, or chilies to taste

1. Warm the bread.
2. Scramble the eggs with the cheese, onion flakes, and salt and pepper.
3. While eggs are cooking, add remaining ingredients.
4. Roll mixture in bread, and then place in microwave on high for 2 minutes.

Prep time 5 min.; cook time 5 min.; beginner skill
435 calories, 32 g protein, 23 g carb, 2 g fiber, 3 g sugar,
26 g fat (11 g saturated fat), 960 mg sodium

CORNBREAD CREPES

16 crepes

>   ¾ cup cornmeal
>   ½ cup brown rice flour
>   ¼ cup oat flour
>   2½ cups buttermilk

¼ cup olive oil
4 large eggs
1 ½ teaspoons salt
1 cup coarsely chopped corn kernels (frozen okay, but
not canned)

1. Combine all ingredients except corn kernels in a blender, and process until smooth.

2. Transfer mixture to bowl, and stir in corn kernels. Cover with plastic wrap. Chill 1 hour.

3. Coat a 7-inch nonstick skillet with vegetable cooking spray; place over medium heat until hot.

4. Pour ¼ cup batter into pan. Quickly tilt pan in all directions so batter covers bottom of pan.

5. Cook one minute, or until top is set. Flip and cook on other side 30 seconds more.

6. Turn out onto wax paper and cool. Repeat with remaining batter.

7. Use with a variety of your favorite fillings to create enchiladas, burritos, savory crepes, etc.

Prep time 5 min + 1 hr. chill, cook time 10 min.; beginner skill
117 calories, 4 g protein, 13 g carb, 1 g fiber, 2 g sugar,
5 g fat (1 g saturated fat), 277 mg sodium

SWEET POTATO WAFFLES (OR PANCAKES)

4 servings

> 8 ounces sweet potatoes, peeled, cooked, and mashed
>   (about ¾ cup)
> 1½ teaspoons olive oil
> 1 large egg white, lightly beaten
> ¾ cup milk (cow, oat, almond, or rice)
> ½ cup brown rice flour
> 1 teaspoon baking powder
> ¼ teaspoon salt

1. Preheat waffle iron.

2. In a large bowl combine the cooked sweet potatoes, oil, egg white, and milk, and beat until well blended. Add flour, baking powder, and salt, and mix until smooth.

3. Spray hot waffle iron with nonstick cooking spray. Cook waffles according to manufacturer's instructions using ¾ cup batter per waffle.

4. Alternatively, drop ½ cup batter onto hot griddle to make pancakes. Cook until bubbles form on surface, about 3 minutes. Flip pancake onto other side, and cook until golden brown.

5. Serve with apple-pear compote.

Prep time 15 min.; cook time 15 min.; learning skill
180 calories, 5 g protein, 32 g carb, 3 g fiber, 10 g sugar,
3 g fat (1 g saturated fat), 249 mg sodium

DUTCH PUFFED PANCAKES

4 servings

> ⅔ cup water
> ¼ cup butter or olive oil

1 cup Kathleen's Baking Mix (page 213)
4 eggs
sweet or savory filling of your choice (see suggestions
   below)

1. Preheat oven to 400°F. Lightly coat a 9-by-12-inch baking pan with cooking spray.
2. Combine water and butter or oil in a medium-size saucepan. Bring to a boil, then add Baking Mix all at once. Stir vigorously over low heat until mixture forms a ball, about 1 minute. Remove from heat.
3. Add eggs, one at a time, beating well after each addition. Batter should be smooth and glossy.
4. Place batter in baking pan—smooth it along the bottom but not up the sides.
5. Bake 30 minutes until puffed and golden.
6. Fill interior of pancake with filling. Serve hot.

Prep time 10 min.; cook time 30 min.; beginner skill
294 calories, 10 g protein, 23 g carb, 2 g fiber, 1 g sugar,
18 g fat (9 g saturated fat), 298 mg sodium

SUGGESTED SAVORY FILLINGS
Chili
Creamed chicken and mushrooms
Roasted garlic vegetables and cheddar cheese
Vegetable chicken stir-fry

SUGGESTED SWEET FILLINGS
Cut fresh seasonal fruits with yogurt or unsweetened
   whipped cream

EASY EGG AND OAT ONE-PAN BREAKFAST

1 serving

> 2 eggs
> ¾ cup milk or yogurt
> 1 cup oats
> 1 small apple, diced
> cinnamon and nutmeg to taste

1. Beat the eggs; stir in milk or yogurt.
2. Add oats, apple, cinnamon, and nutmeg.
3. Cook like a pancake, or scramble in an oiled skillet.

Prep time 5 min.; cook time 5 min.; beginner skill
638 calories, 30 g protein, 84 g carb, 11 g fiber, 26 g sugar,
28 g fat (5 g saturated fat), 222 mg sodium

APPLE HAM BAKE BREAKFAST

6 servings

> 2 cups diced ham
> 2 cups chopped apple, cored but not peeled
> 1½ cups Kathleen's Baking Mix (page 213)
> 1½ cups milk (cow, oat, almond, or rice)
> 4 eggs, lightly beaten
> 2 cups shredded cheddar cheese

1. Heat oven to 375°F. Lightly coat a 9-by-12-inch baking pan with cooking spray.
2. Combine ham and apple, and spread in baking dish.
3. In a medium bowl, combine Baking Mix, milk, and eggs. Pour over ham and apple mixture.
4. Sprinkle with cheese.

5. Bake uncovered 30–35 minutes, or until knife inserted in center comes out clean.

Prep time 10 min.; cook time 35 min.; beginner skill
494 calories, 31 g protein, 32 g carb, 3 g fiber, 8 g sugar,
26 g fat (13 g saturated fat), 451 mg sodium

Note: You can vary the flavor by changing the meat and cheese or adding other ingredients. For example, you could try leftover grilled chicken and Swiss cheese, or bacon and apple with a little cinnamon, or chicken, green chili, and cheese.

SAUSAGE AND EGG BAKE

6 servings

> 1 pound bulk pork or turkey sausage
> 1 cup Kathleen's Baking Mix (page 213)
> 1 cup shredded cheese (cheddar, mozzarella, Monterey jack, Swiss, or a combination)
> 2 cups milk (cow, oat, almond, or rice)
> 6 large eggs, lightly beaten
> 1 teaspoon dry mustard
> ½ teaspoon dry oregano
> ½ teaspoon dried basil
> ½ teaspoon garlic powder
> 1 teaspoon minced, dried onion
> ¼ cup grated Parmesan
> ¼ teaspoon black pepper

1. In a large skillet over medium-high heat, cook sausage until no longer pink. Drain, and place in large bowl.

2. Add remaining ingredients to cooked sausage. Combine well.

3. Pour sausage mix into a 9-by-13-inch baking pan that has been lightly coated with cooking spray. Cover and refrigerate for at least 4 hours but no longer than 24 hours.

4. Heat oven to 350°F. Bake uncovered for 1 hour, or until knife inserted in center comes out clean.

Prep time 15 min + 4 hrs. chill; cook time 60 min.; beginner skill
572 calories, 33 g protein, 22 g carb, 2 g fiber, 6 g sugar,
39 g fat (16 g saturated fat), 1355 mg sodium

LUNCH AND DINNER IDEAS

EASY DOES IT PIZZA

4 servings

1½ cups Kathleen's Baking Mix (page 213)
⅓ cup hot water
1 cup pizza sauce, sugar free
1½ cups shredded mozzarella cheese
½ cup sliced mushrooms
½ cup sliced onions
½ cup sliced peppers
1 cup cooked chicken, cut into strips
½ cup broccoli
½ teaspoon dried basil
½ teaspoon dried oregano
½ teaspoon garlic powder
¼ teaspoon black pepper

1. Heat oven to 450°F. Lightly coat a 12-inch cooking pan with cooking spray.

2. Combine Baking Mix and hot water in a medium-size bowl. Beat until a soft dough forms. Press the dough into a pizza pan. Pinch the edge to form a ½-inch rim.

3. Spread the pizza sauce over the dough. Sprinkle with half the mozzarella cheese. Top with vegetables and chicken.

4. Sprinkle on remaining mozzarella. Season with basil, oregano, garlic powder, and black pepper.

5. Bake 12–15 minutes, or until crust is golden and cheese is melted.

Prep time 15 min.; cook time 15 min.; beginner skill
420 calories, 29 g protein, 46 g carb, 6 g fiber, 6 g sugar,
13 g fat (6 g saturated fat), 666 mg sodium

CHICKEN DRUMMETTES

4 servings

1 cup red pepper sauce
1 teaspoon garlic powder
12 chicken wings, cut in half at joint
2 tablespoons olive oil
1 cup Kathleen's Baking Mix (page 213)
¾ teaspoon onion powder
½ teaspoon black pepper
1 teaspoon dried parsley flakes

1. Combine red pepper sauce and garlic powder. Place chicken in glass baking dish. Pour pepper sauce mixture over chicken, cover, and refrigerate for at least 4 hours but not longer than 24 hours.

2. Heat oven to 450°F. Place oil in large baking pan, large enough to hold wing pieces in a single layer.

3. Combine Baking Mix, onion powder, black pepper, and parsley flakes in a medium-size bowl.

4. Remove chicken from marinade, and discard marinade. Dip chicken pieces in Baking Mix mixture to coat. Place pieces in a single layer in the prepared pan.

5. Bake 25 minutes, then turn the pieces. Bake 20–25 minutes longer or until the chicken is golden and cooked through. Serve hot or cold with blue cheese dressing.

Prep time 10 min + 1 hr. marinade; cook time 60 min.; beginner skill
521 calories, 31 g protein, 26 g carb, 3 g fiber, 2 g sugar,
32 g fat (8 g saturated fat), 241 mg sodium

CURRIED CHICKEN SALAD

4 servings

> 3 cups cooked chicken, cubed
> 3 hard-boiled eggs, chopped
> 1 ½ cups sugar-free mayonnaise
> 1 tablespoon curry powder, or to taste
> ½ teaspoon garlic powder
> ½ cup fresh orange segments
> ½ cup sliced scallions
> ½ cup sliced black olives
> ½ cup chopped cilantro
> ½ cup chopped pecans or almonds
> ¼ teaspoon salt, or to taste
> ¼ teaspoon black pepper, or to taste

Combine all ingredients. Serve immediately, or refrigerate up to 3 days. Good over mixed greens as a main-course salad or as a sandwich filling.

Prep time 30 min.; cook time 0 min.; beginner skill
485 calories, 42 g protein, 11 g carb, 3 g fiber, 5 g sugar,
30 g fat (5 g saturated fat), 656 mg sodium

QUICKIE OVEN-FRIED CHICKEN

4 servings

> *1 tablespoon butter or olive oil*
> *⅔ cup Kathleen's Baking Mix (page 213)*
> *1½ teaspoons paprika*
> *1 teaspoon garlic powder*
> *1¼ teaspoons salt*
> *¼ teaspoon black pepper*
> *3 pounds cut-up broiler-fryer chicken*

1. Heat oven to 425°F. Melt the butter or olive oil in a 9-by-12-inch baking pan.
2. Mix Baking Mix, paprika, garlic powder, salt, and pepper. Coat the chicken in the mixture, and place skin side down in the *hot* prepared pan.
3. Bake uncovered 35 minutes. Turn chicken. Bake about 15 minutes longer, or until the juice of the chicken is not pink when the center of the thickest part is cut.

Prep time 10 min.; cook time 50–60 min.; beginner skill
841 calories, 66 g protein, 16 g carb, 2 g fiber, 0.1 g sugar,
55 g fat (17 g saturated fat), 1074 mg sodium

Note: For Mexican Chicken, decrease Baking Mix to ½ cup; add 2 tablespoons cornmeal and 2 tablespoons chili powder. For Italian Chicken, decrease Baking Mix to ⅓ cup and salt to ½ teaspoon. Add ½ cup grated Parmesan, ½ teaspoon basil, and ½ teaspoon oregano.

EASY CHICKEN BROCCOLI PIE

6 servings

> 2 cups fresh broccoli florets
> 1½ cups shredded cheddar cheese
> 2 cups cooked chicken, cut into strips
> ½ cup red onion, cut into ½-inch dice
> ½ cup Kathleen's Baking Mix (page 213)
> 1 cup milk
> ½ teaspoon salt
> ¼ teaspoon pepper
> ½ teaspoon dried mustard
> 2 eggs, lightly beaten

1. Preheat oven to 400°F. Lightly coat a 9-inch baking pan with cooking oil.

2. Combine broccoli, 1 cup of the cheese, chicken, and onion, and place in prepared pan.

3. Combine the remaining ingredients until well blended, and pour into the pan.

4. Bake 35 minutes, or until a knife inserted in the center comes out clean. Sprinkle with the remaining ½ cup cheese. Return to oven until cheese melts, about 2 minutes. Let stand 5 minutes before serving.

Prep time 15 min.; cook time 35–45 min.; beginner skill
302 calories, 26 g protein, 13 g carb, 1 g fiber, 3 g sugar,
16 g fat (8 g saturated fat), 498 mg sodium

KATHLEEN'S MACARONI AND CHEESE

4 servings

> 8 ounces uncooked brown rice pasta
> 1 ½ cups sharp cheddar cheese, shredded
> 2 ½ cups milk

1. Preheat oven to 350°F.
2. Cook pasta according to directions. Drain well and place in a 1-quart ovenproof mixing bowl.
3. Add cheese to pasta. Combine well.
4. Pour milk over pasta mixture.
5. Bake 35–45 minutes, or until cheese sauce is bubbling and top of mixture is golden brown.

Prep time 5 min.; cook time 45 min.; beginner skill
453 calories, 24 g protein, 47 g carb, 3 g fiber, 9 g sugar,
19 g fat (11 g saturated fat), 422 mg sodium

MACARONI AND CHEESE PIE

6 servings

> 1 cup uncooked brown rice elbow macaroni
> 2 cups cheddar cheese, shredded
> ½ cup Kathleen's Baking Mix (page 213)
> 1 ½ cups milk (cow, oat, almond, or rice)
> ¼ teaspoon red pepper sauce
> 2 eggs, lightly beaten
> ½ teaspoon paprika

1. Heat oven to 400°F. Lightly coat a 9-inch pie plate with cooking spray. Place uncooked brown rice pasta in pie plate. Sprinkle with ¼ cup of the cheese.

2. In a medium bowl, combine Baking Mix, milk, red pepper sauce, and eggs. Pour the mixture over the macaroni.

3. Bake 25–30 minutes, or until a knife inserted in the center comes out clean. Sprinkle with the remaining 1¾ cup cheese, and dust with paprika. Bake 1–2 minutes more, or until cheese is melted. Let stand 5 minutes before serving.

Prep time 10 min.; cook time 30 min.; beginner skill

313 calories, 17 g protein, 24 g carb, 2 g fiber, 4 g sugar,

16 g fat (9 g saturated fat), 351 mg sodium

Note: If you like a crunchy topping on your macaroni and cheese, sprinkle ½ cup crushed Triscuits over the top of the casserole in step 2. Proceed as directed in step 3.

BUTTERNUT SQUASH AND PUMPKIN PANCAKES

4 servings

½ cup pumpkin puree (not pumpkin pie filling)
½ cup cooked butternut squash, mashed
2 eggs, lightly beaten
½ cup milk (cow, oat, almond, or rice)
1 cup oat flour
1 cup brown rice flour
2 teaspoons baking powder
1 teaspoon salt
½ teaspoon ground cinnamon
¼ teaspoon ground cloves
butter or oil for griddle

1. Combine pumpkin puree, squash, eggs, and milk in a medium-size bowl.

2. In a separate bowl, stir together the flours, baking powder, salt, cinnamon, and cloves. Add the dry ingredients to the wet, and mix well.

3. Heat a griddle or skillet over medium-high heat. Lightly coat with butter or oil.

4. Pour ¼ cup of batter per pancake, and cook 2–3 minutes until bubbles form on surface. Flip and continue to cook about 3 minutes more. Serve hot with favorite toppings.

Prep time 15 min.; cook time 15 min.; learning skill
337 calories, 11 g protein, 53 g carb, 7 g fiber, 4 g sugar,
9 g fat (3 g saturated fat), 779 mg sodium

ASIAN ACORN SQUASH
4 servings

> 2 acorn squash, cut in half, seeds and strings removed
> ¼ cup lime juice
> ¼ cup applesauce, unsweetened
> 2 tablespoons tamari
> 1 garlic clove, minced
> 2 tablespoons grated fresh ginger root

1. Preheat oven to 400°F.

2. Place squash halves cut side down in a baking dish filled with ½ inch water. Cook 30–45 minutes depending on size.

3. Remove dish from oven, and turn squash cut side up.

4. In a small bowl, stir together the remaining ingredients. Spoon the mixture into the squash cavities.

5. Return to the oven, and bake 15 more minutes.

Prep time 10 min.; cook time 45–60 min.; beginner skill
105 calories, 3 g protein, 27 g carb, 4 g fiber, 7 g sugar,
0.3 g fat (0.1 g saturated fat), 510 mg sodium

CARROT APPLE BAKE

4 servings

> 1 *pound carrots, peeled, and cut into 1-inch chunks*
> 1 *pound apples, unpeeled, cored, and cut into 1-inch*
> *chunks*
> ½ *cup apple juice*
> 1 *tablespoon olive oil*
> ½ *teaspoon cinnamon, or to taste*
> ½ *cup toasted almonds*

1. Preheat oven to 375°F. Lightly coat a 9-by-12-inch baking pan with cooking spray.

2. Combine all ingredients except almonds, and place in prepared pan.

3. Bake 35–45 minutes, or until carrots and apples are tender and golden brown.

4. Sprinkle with almonds, and serve hot.

Prep time 10 min.; cook time 35–45 min.; beginner skill
279 calories, 6 g protein, 37 g carb, 9 g fiber, 26 g sugar,
14 g fat (2 g saturated fat), 43 mg sodium

ROASTED PEARS AND SQUASH

4 servings

> 3 *cups peeled, cubed squash (butternut, Hubbard, or a*
> *combination of both)*
> 4 *firm Bosc pears, unpeeled, cored, and cut into eighths*

1 cup apple juice, unsweetened
2 tablespoons butter, broken into bits
1 teaspoon cinnamon

1. Preheat oven to 400°F.

2. Lightly coat a 9-by-13-inch baking pan with cooking spray. Combine squash and pears and place in pan.

3. Pour apple juice over mixture. Sprinkle with butter bits and cinnamon.

4. Cover with foil, and bake 25 minutes.

5. Remove foil, bake 30 minutes more, or until pears and squash are tender and golden. Serve hot.

Prep time 10 min.; cook time 45 min.; beginner skill
211 calories, 2 g protein, 41 g carb, 7 g fiber, 24 g sugar,
7 g fat (4 g saturated fat), 65 mg sodium

CRANBERRY-GLAZED ACORN SQUASH
4 servings

3 medium acorn squash (about 1 pound each)
2 cups Cranberry Chutney (see page 219)

1. Preheat oven to 400°F.

2. Cut off the ends of the squash. With a sharp knife, carefully cut each squash crosswise into 4 rings each. Discard the seeds and strings.

3. Place squash rings in a single layer on a large cookie sheet lightly coated with cooking spray. Bake for 15 minutes.

4. Remove squash from oven, and brush ½ Cranberry Chutney onto the surface of each ring. Return to oven, and bake for 20 more minutes.

5. Remove from oven, and brush remaining chutney onto slices. Bake another 15 minutes. Serve hot.

Prep time 5 min.; cook time 60 min.; beginner skill
236 calories, 5 g protein, 48 g carb, 8 g fiber, 19 g sugar,
6 g fat (0.4 g saturated fat), 12 mg sodium

GARLIC ROASTED POTATOES

4 servings

> 4 large potatoes, russet or Yukon gold
> 3 tablespoons olive oil
> ½ teaspoon granulated garlic powder
> salt and pepper to taste
> 2 garlic cloves, minced

1. Preheat oven to 400°F.
2. Scrub potatoes; do not peel. Cut into 2-inch chunks.
3. Toss potatoes with olive oil, garlic powder, salt, and pepper.
4. Place potatoes in lightly oiled baking pan, and bake for 45 minutes, stirring occasionally.
5. Add fresh minced garlic to potatoes, and toss to coat. Return to oven, and bake another 5 minutes until fresh garlic is heated through and potatoes are tender and golden.

Prep time 5 min.; cook time 50 min.; beginner skill
313 calories, 5 g protein, 52 g carb, 5 g fiber, 3 g sugar,
10 g fat (1 g saturated fat), 89 mg sodium

CHEDDAR CHEESE MASHED POTATOES

4 servings

> 4 medium russet potatoes, scrubbed, unpeeled
> ¾ cup sharp cheddar cheese, shredded
> ¼ cup milk (cow, oat, almond, or rice)
> 2 tablespoons fresh chopped herbs of your choice
>   (chives, parsley, chervil, and marjoram all work
>   well, alone or in combination)
> salt and pepper to taste

1. Cut potatoes into 2-inch chunks. Place in medium saucepan, adding enough lightly salted water to cover.

2. Bring to a boil, lower heat, and continue to cook until potatoes are tender, 15–20 minutes. Drain well.

3. Place potatoes in a large mixing bowl. With hand beater or electric mixer, mash them until they are somewhat creamy.

4. Add cheese and milk. Mix just until combined.

5. Add herbs, salt, and pepper. Mix well, and serve hot.

Prep time 5 min.; cook time 25 min.; beginner skill
296 calories, 10 g protein, 48 g carb, 5 g fiber, 4 g sugar,
8 g fat (5 g saturated fat), 228 mg sodium

ROASTED GARLIC MASHED POTATOES

3–4 servings

> 1 head garlic
> 2 teaspoons olive oil
> 6 russet potatoes, scrubbed, unpeeled
> 2 tablespoons butter
> ¼ cup milk
> salt and pepper to taste

1. Preheat oven to 375°F. Slice approximately ¾-inch off the top of the garlic head, just to expose the tops of all the individual cloves. (Do not cut through the root end, because garlic will come apart.) Place the garlic on a square of foil large enough to enclose the entire head. Sprinkle with olive oil, and wrap the foil loosely around the garlic.

2. Bake for 1 hour, or until garlic cloves are very soft and fragrant. Remove from oven, and cool slightly.

3. Cut potatoes into 2-inch chunks. Place in a medium saucepan, adding enough lightly salted water to cover. Bring to a boil, lower heat, and continue to cook until potatoes are tender, 15–20 minutes. Drain well.

4. Place potatoes in a large mixing bowl. Squeeze soft roasted garlic from each of the cloves. The pulp will be very creamy and easily slip out of the skins. Add to potatoes.

5. With a hand beater or electric mixer, mash garlic pulp and potatoes until somewhat creamy.

6. Add butter, milk, salt, and pepper to taste. Combine well and serve hot.

Prep time 15 min.; cook time 60 min.; beginner skill
286 calories, 5 g protein, 49 g carb, 5 g fiber, 4 g sugar,
9 g fat (4 g saturated fat), 154 mg sodium

Note: Roasted garlic stores well in the refrigerator and is a good condiment to have on hand for various soups, stews, dressings, and vegetable preparations. Instead of just roasting 1 head for this recipe alone, purchase 6 or so heads at a time, roast them as directed, and store them unpeeled in plastic bags. If you prefer long-term storage, you can squeeze the pulp from the skins, place it in an airtight plastic bag, and freeze it up to 6 months.

SWEET RUSSET BLUES

4 servings

> 2 *large yams or sweet potatoes, scrubbed, unpeeled*
> 2 *large russet potatoes, scrubbed, unpeeled*
> 6 *medium purple potatoes, scrubbed, unpeeled*
> 3 *tablespoons olive oil*
> 2 *teaspoons garlic powder*
> 1 *tablespoon parsley flakes*
> 1 *teaspoon thyme*
> 1 *teaspoon coriander*
> 1 *teaspoon cumin*
> *salt and freshly cracked pepper to taste*

1. Preheat oven to 400°F.

2. Cut all potatoes into 2-inch chunks. Toss with remaining ingredients, and place in a large baking pan lightly coated with cooking spray.

3. Bake 45–50 minutes, or until potatoes are tender and lightly browned.

Prep time 10 min.; cook time 60 min.; beginner skill
477 calories, 8 g protein, 89 g carb, 9 g fiber, 8 g sugar,
11 g fat (2 g saturated fat), 107 mg sodium

DESSERTS AND SNACKS

APPLE PEAR COMPOTE

6 servings

> 3 *firm pears, peeled, cored, and cut into ½-inch dice*
> 3 *cooking apples, peeled, cored, and cut into ½-inch*
> *dice*
> 1 *teaspoon cinnamon (or more to taste)*
> 1 *teaspoon pure vanilla extract*
> *apple juice, organic, no sugar added*

1. Combine pears, apples, cinnamon, and vanilla in a medium saucepan.
2. Add enough juice to barely cover the top of the fruit.
3. Bring to a boil over high heat. Reduce heat to simmer, and let cook about 20 minutes or until most of the water evaporates and the fruit is soft.
4. Taste, and correct seasonings. Cook before using.

Prep time 15 min.; cook time 20 min.; beginner skill
112 calories, .2 g protein, 28 g carb, 4 g fiber, 22 g sugar,
1 g fat (0 g saturated fat), 1 mg sodium

APPLE PEAR CRISP

6 servings

> 4 *sweet cooking apples (such as Delicious, Rome, or*
> *Gala), peeled, cored, and sliced*
> 3 *firm pears, peeled, cored, and sliced*
> 1½ *cups unsweetened apple juice*
> 2 *teaspoons cinnamon*

2 *tablespoons cornstarch dissolved in ¼ cup apple juice*
1 *teaspoon cinnamon*
1 *cup rolled oats*
½ *cup chopped walnuts or pecans*
1 *tablespoon walnut oil*
2 *tablespoons apple juice*

1. Preheat oven to 350°F. Lightly coat an 8-inch-square baking pan with cooking spray.

2. Combine apples, pears, apple juice, and cinnamon in a large saucepan, and bring to a boil over medium-high heat. Reduce heat, and continue to cook uncovered until fruit is slightly softened but not mushy, about 10 minutes.

3. Raise heat, and bring to a boil. Quickly whisk in cornstarch mixture, and cook until fruit and sauce are thickened. Let cool slightly, then pour into prepared pan.

4. Combine remaining ingredients to form a crumbly mixture. Bake for 25–30 minutes, or until top is golden and fruit is bubbly. Serve warm or at room temperature.

Prep time 15 min.; cook time 45 min.; learning skill
282 calories, 5 g protein, 48 g carb, 6 g fiber, 28 g sugar,
10 g fat (1 g saturated fat), 4 mg sodium

QUICK APPLE COBBLER

4 servings

> 1 21-ounce can sliced apples, packed in water,
>   undrained
> 1 teaspoon cinnamon
> 1 teaspoon vanilla extract
> ½ cup chopped nuts (almonds or walnuts)
> 1 tablespoon cornstarch
> 1 cup Kathleen's Baking Mix (page 213)
> ¼ cup milk (cow, oat, almond, or rice)
> 1 tablespoon softened butter
> ½ teaspoon maple flavoring (optional)

1. Preheat oven to 400°F.

2. Combine apples, cinnamon, vanilla, nuts, and cornstarch. Spread onto an ungreased 8-inch-square baking pan. Place pan in oven and warm apple mixture, about 5 minutes.

3. While apples are warming, combine Baking Mix, milk, butter, and optional maple flavoring to form soft dough. Drop dough onto warmed apples, and return pan to oven.

4. Bake 15–20 minutes, or until topping is golden and apples are hot. Serve with unsweetened whipped cream or yogurt.

Prep time 10 min.; cook time 20 min.; beginner skill
303 calories, 8 g protein, 40 g carb, 6 g fiber, 11 g sugar,
14 g fat (3 g saturated fat), 156 mg sodium

MIXED BERRY COBBLER

6 servings

> 4 cups berries of your choice, fresh or frozen
> 1½ cups apple juice
> ¾ teaspoon cinnamon
> 1 tablespoon cornstarch diluted in 2 tablespoons
>   apple juice
> 1 teaspoon vanilla extract
> 1 recipe Cobbler Crust (page 218)

1. Preheat oven to 375°F.

2. If using frozen berries, let them thaw to a half-frozen state. If using fresh berries, wash them thoroughly and drain well.

3. In a large saucepan, combine berries, apple juice, and cinnamon. Bring to a boil, stirring occasionally to prevent berries from sticking. (Do not overstir, or berries will get mushy.)

4. When the mixture comes to a boil, whisk in cornstarch paste and stir vigorously. Let cook 1–2 minutes, or until nicely thickened. Remove from heat. Stir in vanilla.

5. Pour berry mixture into an 8-inch-square greased baking pan or into individual baking cups. Top with Cobbler Crust.

6. Bake for 25–30 minutes.

Prep time 10 min.; cook time 35–45 min.; beginner skill
152 calories, 3 g protein, 27 g carb, 7 g fiber, 12 g sugar,
4 g fat (2 g saturated fat), 104 mg sodium

PEACH AND BLUEBERRY CRUMBLE

6 servings

> 1 *package frozen blueberries (10 ounces)*
> 2½ *teaspoons cinnamon*
> ¼ *cup plus 2 tablespoons unsweetened apple juice*
> 1 *package frozen peaches (10 ounces) defrosted*
> 1 *tablespoon cornstarch or arrowroot dissolved in*
>   2 *tablespoons apple juice*
> ¼ *cup rolled oats*
> ¼ *cup brown rice flour*
> ¼ *cup chopped walnuts or pecans*
> 2 *tablespoons butter or light olive oil*
> 1 *teaspoon vanilla*

1. Preheat oven to 350°F. Lightly coat an 8-inch-square baking pan with cooking spray.

2. Combine blueberries, 1½ teaspoons of the cinnamon, and ¼ cup of the apple juice in a medium saucepan. Bring to a boil. Add peaches, and combine. Return to boil.

3. When the mixture has returned to boil, add the cornstarch paste. Continue to cook over medium-high heat, stirring constantly until the mixture is thick. Let cool slightly, and then pour into prepared pan.

4. In a small bowl, combine oats, flour, nuts, and the remaining 1 teaspoon cinnamon. Add butter or olive oil, and lightly combine until mixture resembles coarse meal. *Do not* overmix.

5. Add remaining 2 tablespoons apple juice and vanilla. Combine lightly, and sprinkle crumble mixture over prepared blueberry-peach mixture.

6. Bake for about 25 minutes, until golden and bubbly.

Prep time 10 min.; cook time 25–35 min.; beginner skill
167 calories, 2 g protein, 24 g carb, 4 g fiber, 11 g sugar,
8 g fat (3 g saturated fat), 41 mg sodium

BAKED APPLES WITH WALNUT SAUCE

4 servings

> *4 medium baking apples (such as Rome beauty, Fuji,*
> *   Gala, Pippin, or Red Delicious), unpeeled*
> *¾ cup chopped walnuts*
> *1 ½ teaspoons cinnamon*
> *½ teaspoon ground ginger*
> *½ teaspoon ground cloves*
> *1 teaspoon vanilla*
> *1 ½ cups apple juice*
> *2 tablespoons walnut or hazelnut oil (optional)*

1. Preheat oven to 375°F.

2. Wash and core the apples, leaving the peels intact. Place apples in lightly oiled 8-inch-square pan.

3. Toss the walnuts with cinnamon, ginger, and cloves. Press walnut mixture into the center cavities of the cored apples; you will have walnuts left over.

4. Combine remaining walnuts, vanilla, and apple juice, and pour over apples. Sprinkle with optional walnut oil.

5. Cover with aluminum foil, and bake for 45 minutes. Remove foil, and bake 15–20 more minutes, until apples are tender but not mushy.

6. If the walnut sauce is too thin for your liking, pour it into a small saucepan and bring to boil. Lightly thicken with 1 teaspoon cornstarch diluted in 2 teaspoons apple juice. Whisk to combine, and pour over apples.

7. Let apples cool in sauce. They may be served warm or cold with unsweetened whipped cream if so desired.

Prep time 10 min.; cook time 1 hr. + 15 min.; beginner skill
335 calories, 6 g protein, 36 g carb, 6 g fiber, 27 g sugar,
21 g fat (2 g saturated fat), 4 mg sodium

RICE PUDDING WITH APPLES

4 servings

> 1 cup basmati brown rice (or other rice of your choosing)
> 2 cups unsweetened apple juice
> 1 cup apples, peeled, cored, and diced
> 1 teaspoon cinnamon
> 2½ cups milk (cow, oat, almond, or rice)
> 1 teaspoon vanilla

1. Combine rice and juice in a 2-quart saucepan. Cover, and bring to a boil. Reduce to a simmer, and cook until liquid is nearly absorbed, about 20 minutes.

2. Add apples and cinnamon. Stir to combine.

3. Begin adding milk, starting with about ¾ cup, and cook, uncovered, until liquid is absorbed. Continue adding milk as necessary until rice is creamy and thick. Remove from heat.

4. Stir in vanilla. Pour into serving cups and chill at least 2 hours before serving. Sprinkle with additional cinnamon and nutmeg if desired.

5. You can vary this recipe by changing the fruits to your preference. For example, try pears and pear juice, or apricots and apricot juice.

Prep time 10 min.; cook time 75 min.; beginner skill
321 calories, 9 g protein, 63 g carb, 3 g fiber, 25 g sugar,
5 g fat (2 g saturated fat), 84 mg sodium

FRENCH APPLE PIE

8 servings

FOR FILLING

*3 cups sliced apples (Gala, Braeburn, or Fuji work
   well)*
½ cup Kathleen's Baking Mix (page 213)
½ cup apple juice
½ cup milk
1 tablespoon butter, softened
1 teaspoon cinnamon
¼ teaspoon nutmeg
2 eggs, lightly beaten

FOR STREUSEL TOPPING

½ cup Kathleen's Baking Mix
¼ cup chopped nuts
¼ cup rolled oats
1 teaspoon vanilla extract
1 teaspoon cinnamon
2 tablespoons butter, cut into small bits

1. Preheat oven to 350°F. Lightly coat a 9-inch pie pan
with cooking spray.

2. Combine streusel topping ingredients in a small
bowl—mixture should be crumbly. Set aside.

3. Spread apples in bottom of pie pan.

4. Combine remaining pie ingredients in a medium-size bowl until well blended. Pour over apples. Sprinkle with streusel topping.

5. Bake 40–45 minutes, or until a knife inserted in the center comes out clean. Cool 5 minutes before serving. Serve with yogurt or unsweetened whipped cream.

Prep time 15 min.; cook time 45 min.; beginner skill
192 calories, 5 g protein, 23 g carb, 3 g fiber, 8 g sugar,
9 g fat (4 g saturated fat), 127 mg sodium

APPLE PIE WITH CHEDDAR CRUST

1 9-inch pie (6–8 servings)

FOR CRUST

1 cup oat or brown rice flour, or a combination of both
½ teaspoon baking powder
¼ teaspoon salt
3 tablespoons cold butter
2 tablespoons Crisco or other solid vegetable shortening
⅓ cup ice water
1 cup shredded sharp cheddar cheese

FOR FILLING

2½ pounds apples, peeled, cored, and sliced
2 cups unsweetened apple juice
½ teaspoon cinnamon
1 tablespoon cornstarch dissolved in 2 tablespoons
  apple juice
½ teaspoon vanilla

FOR CRUST

1. In a medium bowl combine flour, baking powder, and salt with pastry blender or 2 knives. Cut in butter and shortening until mixture forms coarse crumbs.

2. Stir in ice water just until dough comes together. Stir in cheese, and combine well.

3. Form dough into a disk, and wrap in plastic wrap. Refrigerate 1 hour.

FOR FILLING

1. Combine apples, juice, and cinnamon in a large saucepan. Bring to a boil.

2. Once the apple mixture boils, lower heat to simmer, and cook 10–15 minutes.

3. Return to boil, and thicken by adding cornstarch mixture. Remove from heat, and let cool slightly. Stir in vanilla.

TO ASSEMBLE

1. Preheat oven to 450°F. Spoon the apple mixture into 9-inch pie pan sprayed with nonstick cooking spray.

2. On a lightly floured surface, quickly roll out the crust into a 13-inch round. Drape the crust over the apples, and crimp the edges to seal. With a sharp knife, cut 2 or 3 slits in the dough for steam vents.

3. Set the pie pan on a baking sheet, and place in the oven. Bake 20 minutes. Reduce oven temperature to 350°F and bake 15 minutes more, or until crust is golden and apples are tender. Let cool at least ½ hour before cutting.

Prep time 20 min. + 1 hr. chill; cook time 35–45 min.; experienced skill
395 calories, 7 g protein, 56 g carb, 5 g fiber, 33 g sugar,
18 g fat (8 g saturated fat), 293 mg sodium

PUMPKIN PECAN PIE

8 servings

FOR FILLING

1 cup canned pumpkin (not pumpkin pie filling)
1 cup evaporated milk
½ cup Kathleen's Baking Mix (page 213)
⅓ cup apple juice concentrate
½ teaspoon maple flavoring
1 tablespoon butter, softened
1 ½ teaspoons pumpkin pie spice
1 teaspoon vanilla
3 eggs, lightly beaten
¾ cup chopped pecans

TOPPING

2 cups heavy cream
1 ½ teaspoons vanilla
½ teaspoon pumpkin pie spice

1. Preheat oven to 350°F. Lightly coat a 9-inch pie pan with cooking spray.

2. Combine all filling ingredients except pecans, and stir until well blended. Add pecans and mix well. Pour into prepared pie pan.

3. Bake 35–40 minutes, or until a knife inserted in the center comes out clean. Cool completely before slicing. Serve with topping.

4. To prepare topping, beat heavy cream with an electric mixer at high speed until very thick and just beginning to peak. Add vanilla and pie spice, and continue to beat until cream is stiff and holds a peak.

Prep time 10 min.; cook time 35–40 min.; beginner skill
425 calories, 8 g protein, 20 g carb, 2 g fiber, 11 g sugar,
36 g fat (17 g saturated fat), 125 mg sodium

BERRY SHORTCAKES

6 servings

> 1½ *cups Kathleen's Baking Mix (page 213)*
> 6 *tablespoons melted butter*
> 1 *cup milk (cow, oat, almond, or rice)*
> ½ *teaspoon vanilla or almond extract*
> ½ *teaspoon cinnamon*
> ¼ *teaspoon nutmeg*
> 4 *cups berries of your choice*
> 1 *cup unsweetened whipped cream*

1. Preheat oven to 425°F.

2. Combine all ingredients except berries and cream in a medium-size bowl until a soft dough forms. Do not overmix.

3. Drop dough by large spoonfuls onto ungreased cookie sheet.

4. Bake 10–12 minutes, or until golden brown. Remove from oven, and cool slightly.

5. Split warm shortcakes, and fill with berries and cream.

Prep time 10 min.; cook time 15 min.; beginner skill
350 calories, 6 g protein, 35 g carb, 8 g fiber, 7 g sugar,
21 g fat (12 g saturated fat), 263 mg sodium

BLUEBERRY CREAM PARFAIT

6 servings

> 1 *pound frozen blueberries*
> ¼ *cup unsweetened apple juice*
> 1 *tablespoon cornstarch or arrowroot dissolved in*
>   2 *tablespoons apple juice or water*
> 1–2 *teaspoons cinnamon (according to taste)*
> 8 *ounces cream cheese (reduced fat or no fat is okay)*
> 1 *recipe Rice Pudding with Apples (page 246), chilled*

1. Combine blueberries, apple juice, and cornstarch mixture and 1 teaspoon of the cinnamon in a 2-quart saucepan. Bring to a boil over high heat.

2. When mixture is cooled, scrape into a blender. Add cream cheese, and blend until mixture is uniform and creamy. Taste, and add additional cinnamon if desired.

3. Assemble parfaits in parfait glasses or some other pretty, clear serving pieces of your choice. Make several layers by alternating the blueberry mixture and the rice pudding. Dust the top with additional cinnamon and/or nutmeg if desired. Chill at least 2 hours before serving.

Prep time 30 min.; cook time 60 min.; experienced skill
393 calories, 8 g protein, 59 g carb, 4 g fiber, 27 g sugar,
16 g fat (9 g saturated fat), 164 mg sodium

CAROB OATMEAL COOKIES

12 dozen (36 servings of 4 cookies each)

> 3 *cups mashed bananas*
> 2 *cups vegetable oil*
> 1 ½ *teaspoons vanilla extract*

1 dozen large eggs
1½ cups milk
7½ cups whole wheat or oat flour
1½ cups carob powder
1½ teaspoons baking soda
6 cups chopped walnuts
4 cups rolled oats

1. Preheat oven to 350°F.

2. In a large mixing bowl, beat together mashed bananas, oil, vanilla, eggs, and milk until creamy.

3. Add flour, carob powder, and baking soda. Beat well.

4. Stir in walnuts and oats. Mix well.

5. Drop batter by small teaspoonfuls onto oiled baking sheets.

6. Bake for 8 to 10 minutes, or until just firm to touch. Cool on wire racks.

Prep time 10 min.; cook time 10 min.; beginner skill
443 calories, 9 g protein, 35 g carb, 8 g fiber, 4 g sugar,
30 g fat (4 g saturated fat), 90 mg sodium

HOMEMADE TRAIL MIX

8 servings (basic recipe)

1 cup almonds
1 cup rolled oats
½ cup sunflower seeds
½ cup pumpkin seeds
½ cup unsweetened coconut, flaked and dried
1 cup unsweetened puffed brown rice cereal
3 tablespoons olive oil

OPTIONAL FLAVORINGS

1 teaspoon cumin
1 teaspoon chili powder

1 teaspoon vanilla
1 ½ teaspoons cinnamon

1 teaspoon almond extract
½ teaspoon coconut extract

1 teaspoon maple flavoring
1 teaspoon cinnamon

(omit coconut)
1 tablespoon Parmesan cheese
1 teaspoon garlic powder

(omit coconut)
1 ½ teaspoons tamari
¼ teaspoon ground ginger
½ teaspoon garlic powder

1. Preheat oven to 350°F.

2. Combine trail mix ingredients in a large bowl. Add flavorings if desired.

3. Spread mixture on a cookie sheet lightly coated with cooking spray.

4. Bake 15 minutes, stirring frequently, until ingredients are golden brown and flavors are set.

Prep time 10 min.; cook time 15 min.; beginner skill
354 calories, 6 g protein, 17 g carb, 7 g fiber, 3 g sugar,
26 g fat (4 g saturated fat), 15 mg sodium (basic recipe only)

RESOURCES

We offer a number of resources for you online. Please visit our website at www.radiantrecovery.com or our site for children at www.radiantkids.com.

You can sign up for our free newsletter, join our community forum, or join one of our online support groups. Of particular interest may be the list for parents, teens, or kids.

You may purchase George's Shake or George's Junior from our online store at www.radiantrecoverystore.com.

Kathleen also does private consultations. More information may be found at www.radiantrecovery.com or by calling 1 (888) 579-3970.

You may contact Kathleen by writing her at kathleen@radiantrecovery.com.

BIBLIOGRAPHY

Anderson, C. A., and B. J. Bushman (2001). "Effects of violent video games on aggressive behavior, aggressive cognition, aggressive affect, physiological arousal, and prosocial behavior: a meta-analytic review of the scientific literature." *Psychol Sci* 12(5): 353–9.

Appelbaum, B. D., and S. G. Holtzman (1984). "Characterization of stress-induced potentiation of opioid effects in the rat." *J Pharmacol Exp Ther* 231(3): 555–65.

Avena, N. M., and B. G. Hoebel (2003). "Amphetamine-sensitized rats show sugar-induced hyperactivity (cross-sensitization) and sugar hyperphagia." *Pharmacol Biochem Behav* 74(3): 635–9.

Bachmanov, A. A., D. R. Reed, et al. (1997). "Sucrose consumption in mice: major influence of two genetic loci affecting peripheral sensory responses." *Mamm Genome* 8(8): 545–8.

Bachmanov, A. A., M. G. Tordoff, et al. (1996). "Ethanol consumption and taste preferences in C57BL/6ByJ and 129/J mice." *Alcohol Clin Exp Res* 20(2): 201–6.

Baird, D. D., D. M. Umbach, et al. (1995). "Dietary intervention study to assess estrogenicity of dietary soy among postmenopausal women." *J Clin Endocrinol Metab* 80(5): 1685–90.

Bernstein, G. A., M. E. Carroll, et al. (2002). "Caffeine dependence in teenagers." *Drug Alcohol Depend* 66(1): 1–6.

Birch, L. L., L. McPhee, et al. (1989). "Children's food intake following drinks sweetened with sucrose or aspartame: time course effects." *Physiol Behav* 45(2): 387–95.

Biver, F., F. Lotstra, et al. (1996). "Sex difference in 5HT2 receptor in the living human brain." *Neurosci Lett* 204(1–2): 25–8.

Blass, E., E. Fitzgerald, et al. (1987). "Interactions between sucrose, pain and isolation distress." *Pharmacol Biochem Behav* 26(3): 483–9.

Blass, E. M. (1996). "Mothers and their infants: peptide-mediated physiological, behavioral and affective changes during suckling." *Regul Pept* 66(1–2): 109–12.

Blass, E. M., and L. B. Hoffmeyer (1991). "Sucrose as an analgesic for newborn infants." *Pediatrics* 87(2): 215–8.

Blass, E. M., and A. Shah (1995). "Pain-reducing properties of sucrose in human newborns." *Chem Senses* 20(1): 29–35.

Blass, E. M., and D. J. Shide (1994). "Some comparisons among the calming and pain-relieving effects of sucrose, glucose, fructose and lactose in infant rats." *Chem Senses* 19(3): 239–49.

Boyd, J. J., I. Contreras, et al. (1990). "Effect of a high-fat-sucrose diet on in vivo insulin receptor kinase activation." *Am J Physiol* 259(1 Pt. 1): E111–6.

Breneman, J. C. (1959). "Allergic cystitis: the cause of nocturnal enuresis." *Gp* 20: 84–98.

Butchko, H. H., W. W. Stargel, et al. (2002). "Aspartame: review of safety." *Regul Toxicol Pharmacol* 35(2 Pt. 2): S1–93.

Caldarone, B. J., T. P. George, et al. (2000). "Gender differences in learned helplessness behavior are influenced by genetic background." *Pharmacol Biochem Behav* 66(4): 811–7.

Cassidy, A., S. Bingham, et al. (1995). "Biological effects of iso-flavones in young women: importance of the chemical composition of soyabean products." *Br J Nutr* 74(4): 587–601.

Castellanos, F. X., and J. L. Rapoport (2002). "Effects of caffeine on development and behavior in infancy and childhood: a review of the published literature." *Food Chem Toxicol* 40(9): 1235–42.

Christie, M. J., and G. B. Chesher (1982). "Physical dependence on physiologically released endogenous opiates." *Life Sci* 30(14): 1173–7.

Clementz, G. L., and J. W. Dailey (1988). "Psychotropic effects of caffeine." *Am Fam Physician* 37(5): 167–72.

Colantuoni, C., P. Rada, et al. (2002). "Evidence that intermittent, excessive sugar intake causes endogenous opioid dependence." *Obes Res* 10(6): 478–88.

Colantuoni, C., J. Schwenker, et al. (2001). "Excessive sugar intake alters binding to dopamine and mu-opioid receptors in the brain." *Neuroreport* 12(16): 3549–52.

De Waele, J. P., and C. Gianoulakis (1997). "Characterization of the mu and delta opioid receptors in the brain of the C57BL/6 and DBA/2 mice, selected for their differences in voluntary ethanol consumption." *Alcohol Clin Exp Res* 21(4): 754–62.

De Waele, J. P., D. N. Papachristou, et al. (1992). "The alcohol-preferring C57BL/6 mice present an enhanced sensitivity of the hypothalamic beta-endorphin system to ethanol than the alcohol-avoiding DBA/2 mice." *J Pharmacol Exp Ther* 261(2): 788–94.

Divi, R. L., H. C. Chang, et al. (1997). "Anti-thyroid isoflavones from soybean: isolation, characterization, and mechanisms of action." *Biochem Pharmacol* 54(10): 1087–96.

Dray, A., and R. Metsch (1984). "Opioid receptor subtypes involved in the central inhibition of urinary bladder motility." *Eur J Pharmacol* 104(1–2): 47–53.

Dray, A., and L. Nunan (1987). "Mu and delta opioid ligands inhibit reflex contractions of the urinary bladder in the rat by different central mechanisms." *Neuropharmacology* 26(7A): 753–9.

Drewnowski, A. (1987). "Changes in mood after carbohydrate consumption." *Am J Clin Nutr* 46(4): 703–5.

Elliott, S. S., N. L. Keim, et al. (2002). "Fructose, weight gain, and the insulin resistance syndrome." *Am J Clin Nutr* 76(5): 911–22.

Fernstrom, J. D., and R. J. Wurtman (1974). "Control of brain serotonin levels by the diet." *Adv Biochem Psychopharmacol* 11(0): 133–42.

———— (1997). "Brain serotonin content: physiological regulation by plasma neutral amino acids. 1971." *Obes Res* 5(4): 377–80.

Fleetwood, S. W., and S. G. Holtzman (1989). "Stress-induced potentiation of morphine-induced analgesia in morphine-tolerant rats." *Neuropharmacology* 28(6): 563–7.

Funk, J. B., D. D. Buchman, et al. (2000). "Preference for violent electronic games, self-concept, and gender differences in young children." *Am J Orthopsychiatry* 70(2): 233–41.

Giammattei, J., G. Blix, et al. (2003). "Television watching and soft drink consumption: associations with obesity in 11- to 13-year-old schoolchildren." *Arch Pediatr Adolesc Med* 157(9): 882–6.

Gianoulakis, C. (1996). "Implications of endogenous opioids and dopamine in alcoholism: human and basic science studies." *Alcohol Alcohol Suppl* 1: 33–42.

———— (2001). "Influence of the endogenous opioid system on high alcohol consumption and genetic predisposition to alcoholism." *J Psychiatry Neurosci* 26(4): 304–18.

Gianoulakis, C., X. Dai, et al. (2003). "Effect of Chronic Alcohol Consumption on the Activity of the Hypothalamic-Pituitary-Adrenal Axis and Pituitary Beta-Endorphin as a Function of Alcohol Intake, Age, and Gender." *Alcohol Clin Exp Res* 27(3): 410–23.

Gianoulakis, C., and A. Gupta (1986). "Inbred strains of mice with variable sensitivity to ethanol exhibit differences in the content and processing of beta-endorphin." *Life Sci* 39(24): 2315–25.

Giorgetti, R., A. Bussolini, et al. (1996). "[Diabetes and celiac disease: a study related to the association of the two pathologies]." *Minerva Pediatr* 48(3): 85–8.

Gray, L., L. W. Miller, et al. (2002). "Breastfeeding is analgesic in healthy newborns." *Pediatrics* 109(4): 590–3.

Gray, L., L. Watt, et al. (2000). "Skin-to-skin contact is analgesic in healthy newborns." *Pediatrics* 105(1): e14.

Heled, Y., Y. Shapiro, et al. (2002). "Physical exercise prevents the development of type 2 diabetes mellitus in Psammomys obesus." *Am J Physiol Endocrinol Metab* 282(2): E370–5.

——— (2003). "Physical exercise enhances protein kinase C delta activity and insulin receptor tyrosine phosphorylation in diabetes-prone psammomys obesus." *Metabolism* 52(8): 1028–33.

Helm, K. A., P. Rada, et al. (2003). "Cholecystokinin combined with serotonin in the hypothalamus limits accumbens dopamine release while increasing acetylcholine: a possible satiation mechanism." *Brain Res* 963(1–2): 290–7.

Hernanz, A., and I. Polanco (1991). "Plasma precursor amino acids of central nervous system monoamines in children with coeliac disease." *Gut* 32(12): 1478–81.

Herrera, R., G. Manjarrez, et al. (2003). "Serotonin-related tryptophan in children with insulin-dependent diabetes." *Pediatr Neurol* 28(1): 20–3.

Hoebel, B. G. (1997). "Neuroscience and appetitive behavior research: 25 years." *Appetite* 29(2): 119–33.

Holt, S. H., J. C. Miller, et al. (1995). "A satiety index of common foods." *Eur J Clin Nutr* 49(9): 675–90.

Hoza, B., D. A. Waschbusch, et al. (2000). "Attention-deficit/ hyperactivity disordered and control boys' responses to social success and failure." *Child Dev* 71(2): 432–46.

Irvine, C. H., M. G. Fitzpatrick, et al. (1998). "Phytoestrogens in soy-based infant foods: concentrations, daily intake, and possible biological effects." *Proc Soc Exp Biol Med* 217(3): 247–53.

Jamensky, N. T., and C. Gianoulakis (1997). "Content of dynorphins and kappa-opioid receptors in distinct brain regions of C57BL/6 and DBA/2 mice." *Alcohol Clin Exp Res* 21(8): 1455–64.

Kalb, C. (2000). "Drugged-out toddlers. A new study documents an alarming increase in behavior-altering medication for preschoolers." *Newsweek* 135(10): 53.

Kampov-Polevoy, A., J. C. Garbutt, et al. (1997). "Evidence of preference for a high-concentration sucrose solution in alcoholic men." *Am J Psychiatry* 154(2): 269–70.

——— (1999). "Association between preference for sweets and excessive alcohol intake: a review of animal and human studies." *Alcohol Alcohol* 34(3): 386–95.

Kanarek, R. B., W. F. Mathes, et al. (1996). "Intake of dietary sucrose or fat reduces amphetamine drinking in rats." *Pharmacol Biochem Behav* 54(4): 719–23.

Kimmel, H. L., and S. G. Holtzman (1997). "Mu opioid agonists potentiate amphetamine- and cocaine-induced rotational behavior in the rat." *J Pharmacol Exp Ther* 282(2): 734–46.

Klassen, A., A. Miller, et al. (1999). "Attention-deficit hyperactivity disorder in children and youth: a quantitative systematic review of the efficacy of different management strategies." *Can J Psychiatry* 44(10): 1007–16.

Knowles, P. A., R. L. Conner, et al. (1989). "Opiate effects on social behavior of juvenile dogs as a function of social deprivation." *Pharmacol Biochem Behav* 33(3): 533–7.

Kohen-Avramoglu, R., A. Theriault, et al. (2003). "Emergence of the metabolic syndrome in childhood: an epidemiological overview and mechanistic link to dyslipidemia." *Clin Biochem* 36(6): 413–20.

Korponay-Szabo, I. R., J. B. Kovacs, et al. (1999). "High

prevalence of silent celiac disease in preschool children screened with IgA/IgG antiendomysium antibodies." *J Pediatr Gastroenterol Nutr* 28(1): 26–30.

Kruesi, M. J., J. L. Rapoport, et al. (1987). "Effects of sugar and aspartame on aggression and activity in children." *Am J Psychiatry* 144(11): 1487–90.

Leibowitz, S. F., N. M. Avena, et al. (2003). "Ethanol intake increases galanin mRNA in the hypothalamus and withdrawal decreases it." *Physiol Behav* 79(1): 103–11.

Leventhal, L., T. C. Kirkham, et al. (1995). "Selective actions of central mu and kappa opioid antagonists upon sucrose intake in sham-fed rats." *Brain Res* 685(1–2): 205–10.

Lorch, E. P., R. P. Sanchez, et al. (1999). "The relation of story structure properties to recall of television stories in young children with attention-deficit hyperactivity disorder and nonreferred peers." *J Abnorm Child Psychol* 27(4): 293–309.

Markus, C. R., B. Olivier, et al. (2002). "Whey protein rich in alpha-lactalbumin increases the ratio of plasma tryptophan to the sum of the other large neutral amino acids and improves cognitive performance in stress-vulnerable subjects." *Am J Clin Nutr* 75(6): 1051–6.

Martinez, F. J., R. A. Rizza, et al. (1994). "High-fructose feeding elicits insulin resistance, hyperinsulinism, and hypertension in normal mongrel dogs." *Hypertension* 23(4): 456–63.

McGuire, W. J., and C. V. McGuire (1996). "Enhancing self-esteem by directed-thinking tasks: cognitive and affective positivity asymmetries." *J Pers Soc Psychol* 70(6): 1117–25.

Melchior, J. C., D. Rigaud, et al. (1994). "Palatability of a meal influences release of beta-endorphin, and of potential regulators of food intake in healthy human subjects." *Appetite* 22(3): 233–44.

Miczek, K. A., M. L. Thompson, et al. (1982). "Opioid-like analgesia in defeated mice." *Science* 215(4539): 1520–2.

Milich, R., and W. E. Pelham (1986). "Effects of sugar ingestion on the classroom and playground behavior of attention deficit disordered boys." *J Consult Clin Psychol* 54(5): 714–8.

Miller, A. R., C. E. Lalonde, et al. (2001). "Prescription of methylphenidate to children and youth, 1990–1996." *Cmaj* 165(11): 1489–94.

Mohn, A., M. Cerruto, et al. (2001). "Celiac disease in children and adolescents with type I diabetes: importance of hypoglycemia." *J Pediatr Gastroenterol Nutr* 32(1): 37–40.

Moles, A., and S. J. Cooper (1995). "Opioid modulation of sucrose intake in CD-1 mice: effects of gender and housing conditions." *Physiol Behav* 58(4): 791–6.

Morley, J. E., and A. S. Levine (1982). "The role of the endogenous opiates as regulators of appetite." *Am J Clin Nutr* 35(4): 757–61.

Nishizawa, S., C. Benkelfat, et al. (1997). "Differences between males and females in rates of serotonin synthesis in human brain." *Proc Natl Acad Sci U S A* 94(10): 5308–13.

Palmer, L. K. (1995). "Effects of a walking program on attributional style, depression, and self-esteem in women." *Percept Mot Skills* 81(3 Pt. 1): 891–8.

Panksepp, J., R. Meeker, et al. (1980). "The neurochemical control of crying." *Pharmacol Biochem Behav* 12(3): 437–43.

Rada, P., A. Mendialdua, et al. (2003). "Extracellular glutamate increases in the lateral hypothalamus during meal initiation, and GABA peaks during satiation: microdialysis measurements every 30 s." *Behav Neurosci* 117(2): 222–7.

Rada, P., S. A. Moreno, et al. (2003). "Glutamate release in the nucleus accumbens is involved in behavioral depression during the PORSOLT swim test." *Neuroscience* 119(2): 557–65.

Reid, L. D., P. W. Marinelli, et al. (2002). "One injection of estradiol valerate induces dramatic changes in rats' intake of alcoholic beverages." *Pharmacol Biochem Behav* 72(3): 601–16.

Robinson, T. N. (1998). "Does television cause childhood obesity?" *Jama* 279(12): 959–60.

—— (2001). "Television viewing and childhood obesity." *Pediatr Clin North Am* 48(4): 1017–25.

Rushton, J. L., and J. T. Whitmire (2001). "Pediatric stimulant and selective serotonin reuptake inhibitor prescription trends: 1992 to 1998." *Arch Pediatr Adolesc Med* 155(5): 560–5.

Safer, D. J. (2000). "Are stimulants overprescribed for youths with ADHD?" *Ann Clin Psychiatry* 12(1): 55–62.

Sheslow, D., S. Hassink, et al. (1993). "The relationship between self-esteem and depression in obese children." *Ann N Y Acad Sci* 699: 289–91.

Shi, D., O. Nikodijevic, et al. (1994). "Effects of chronic caffeine on adenosine, dopamine and acetylcholine systems in mice." *Arch Int Pharmacodyn Ther* 328(3): 261–87.

Shide, D. J., and E. M. Blass (1991). "Opioid mediation of odor preferences induced by sugar and fat in 6-day-old rats." *Physiol Behav* 50(5): 961–6.

Spangler, R., N. L. Goddard, et al. (2003). "Elevated D3 dopamine receptor mRNA in dopaminergic and dopaminoceptive regions of the rat brain in response to morphine." *Brain Res Mol Brain Res* 111(1–2): 74–83.

Spiers, P. A., L. Sabounjian, et al. (1998). "Aspartame: neuropsychologic and neurophysiologic evaluation of acute and chronic effects." *Am J Clin Nutr* 68(3): 531–7.

Surwit, R. S., M. N. Feinglos, et al. (1995). "Differential effects of fat and sucrose on the development of obesity and diabetes in C57BL/6J and A/J mice." *Metabolism* 44(5): 645–51.

Surwit, R. S., C. M. Kuhn, et al. (1988). "Diet-induced type II diabetes in C57BL/6J mice." *Diabetes* 37(9): 1163–7.

Surwit, R. S., and M. S. Schneider (1993). "Role of stress in the etiology and treatment of diabetes mellitus." *Psychosom Med* 55(4): 380–93.

Thompson, M. L., K. A. Miczek, et al. (1988). "Analgesia in defeated mice: evidence for mediation via central rather than pituitary or adrenal endogenous opioid peptides." *Pharmacol Biochem Behav* 29(3): 451–6.

Tou, J. C., J. Chen, et al. (1998). "Flaxseed and its lignan precursor, secoisolariciresinol diglycoside, affect pregnancy outcome and reproductive development in rats." *J Nutr* 128(11): 1861–8.

Van der Kolk, B. A. (1994). "The body keeps the score: memory and the evolving psychobiology of posttraumatic stress." *Harv Rev Psychiatry* 1(5): 253–65.

Vanderschuren, L. J., R. J. Niesink, et al. (1995). "Mu- and kappa-opioid receptor-mediated opioid effects on social play in juvenile rats." *Eur J Pharmacol* 276(3): 257–66.

Villani, S. (2001). "Impact of media on children and adolescents: a 10-year review of the research." *J Am Acad Child Adolesc Psychiatry* 40(4): 392–401.

Wake, M., K. Hesketh, et al. (2003). "Television, computer use and body mass index in Australian primary school children." *J Paediatr Child Health* 39(2): 130–4.

Witt, P. (1971) "Drugs alter web-building of spiders, a review and evaluation." *Behavior Sci* 16: 98–113

Wolinsky, T. D., K. D. Carr, et al. (1994). "Effects of chronic food restriction on mu and kappa opioid binding in rat forebrain: a quantitative autoradiographic study." *Brain Res* 656(2): 274–80.

Wolraich, M., R. Milich, et al. (1985). "Effects of sucrose ingestion on the behavior of hyperactive boys." *J Pediatr* 106(4): 675–82.

Wolraich, M. L., P. J. Stumbo, et al. (1986). "Dietary characteristics of hyperactive and control boys." *J Am Diet Assoc* 86(4): 500–4.

Wolraich, M. L., D. B. Wilson, et al. (1995). "The effect of sugar on behavior or cognition in children. A meta-analysis." *JAMA* 274(20): 1617–21.

Wurtman, R. J., and J. J. Wurtman (1995). "Brain serotonin, carbohydrate-craving, obesity and depression." *Obes Res* 3, Suppl. 4: 477S–480S.

———— (1996). "Brain serotonin, carbohydrate-craving, obesity and depression." *Adv Exp Med Biol* 398: 35–41.

Zito, J. M., D. J. Safer, et al. (2000). "Trends in the prescribing of psychotropic medications to preschoolers." *JAMA* 283(8): 1025–30.

Zorrilla, E. P., R. J. DeRubeis, et al. (1995). "High self-esteem, hardiness and affective stability are associated with higher basal pituitary-adrenal hormone levels." *Psychoneuroendocrinology* 20(6): 591–601.

INDEX

ABOUT THE AUTHOR

KATHLEEN DESMAISONS, Ph.D., pioneered the field of addictive nutrition with her groundbreaking work in the area of sugar sensitivity and addiction. She is the author of the bestselling *Potatoes Not Prozac, The Sugar Addict's Total Recovery Program,* and *Your Last Diet.* In response to the increasing number of children with behavioral problems, learning struggles, and weight concerns, Dr. DesMaisons created a cutting-edge program to help kids and parents make the nutritional changes that heal sugar sensitive children—and profoundly impact their lives. In her more than thirty years of experience in working with addicts of all ages, Dr. DesMaisons brings the wisdom, compassion, and charm that has given kids around the world a new lens through which they can understand their attraction to and use of sugar and become healthier, end their mood swings, and reverse their low self-esteem. Dr. DesMaisons lives in Albuquerque, New Mexico.